America's Health Care SAFETY NET

Intact but Endangered

Committee on the Changing Market, Managed Care, and the
Future Viability of Safety Net Providers

Marion Ein Lewin and Stuart Altman, *Editors*

INSTITUTE OF MEDICINE

NATIONAL ACADEMY PRESS
Washington, D.C.

NATIONAL ACADEMY PRESS • 2101 Constitution Avenue, N.W. • Washington, D 20418

NOTICE: The project that is the subject of this report was approved by the Governing Board of the National Research Council, whose members are drawn from the councils of the National Academy of Sciences, the National Academy of Engineering, and the Institute of Medicine. The members of the committee responsible for the report were chosen for their special competences and with regard for appropriate balance.

Support for this project was provided by the Health Resources and Services Administration (Contract No. 240-97-0030). The views presented in this report are those of the Institute of Medicine Committee on the Changing Market, Managed Care, and the Future Viability of Safety Net Providers and are not necessarily those of the funding agency.

Library of Congress Cataloging-in-Publication Data

America's health care safety net : intact but endangered / Committee on the Changing Market, Managed Care, and the Future Viability of Safety Net Providers ; Marion Ein Lewin and Stuart Altman, editors.
    p. ; cm
Includes bibliograpical references and index.
ISBN 0-309-06497-X (hardcover)
    1. Medical assistance—United States. 2. Medical care—Needs assessment—United States. 3. Medically uninsured—United States. 4. Poor—Medical care—United States. I. Lewin, Marion Ein. II. Altman, Stuart H. III. Institute of Medicine (U.S.). Committee on the Changing Market, Managed Care, and the Future Viability of Safety Net Providers.
    [DNLM: 1. Medical Assistance—United States. 2. Delivery of Health Care—United States. 3. Medically Uninsured—United States.
W 250 AA1 A512 2000]
RA 395.A3 A5965 2000
362.1'0973—dc21   00-033231

Additional copies of this report are available for sale from the National Academy Press, 2101 Constitution Avenue, N.W., Box 285, Washington, DC 20055. Call (800) 624-6242 or (202) 334-3313 (in the Washington metropolitan area), or visit the NAP's home page at **www.nap.edu**. The full text of this report is available at **www.nap.edu**.

For more information about the Institute of Medicine, visit the IOM home page at **www.iom.edu**.

The serpent has been a symbol of long life, healing, and knowledge among almost all cultures and religions since the beginning of recorded history. The serpent adopted as a logotype by the Institute of Medicine is a relief carving from ancient Greece, now held by the Staatliche Museen in Berlin.

*"Knowing is not enough; we must apply.
Willing is not enough; we must do."*
—Goethe

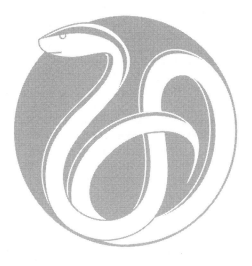

INSTITUTE OF MEDICINE

Shaping the Future for Health

THE NATIONAL ACADEMIES

National Academy of Sciences
National Academy of Engineering
Institute of Medicine
National Research Council

The *National Academy of Sciences* is a private, nonprofit, self-perpetuating society of distinguished scholars engaged in scientific and engineering research, dedicated to the furtherance of science and technology and to their use for the general welfare. Upon the authority of the charter granted to it by the Congress in 1863, the Academy has a mandate that requires it to advise the federal government on scientific and technical matters. Dr. Bruce M. Alberts is president of the National Academy of Sciences.

The **National Academy of Engineering** was established in 1964, under the charter of the National Academy of Sciences, as a parallel organization of outstanding engineers. It is autonomous in its administration and in the selection of its members, sharing with the National Academy of Sciences the responsibility for advising the federal government. The National Academy of Engineering also sponsors engineering programs aimed at meeting national needs, encourages education and research, and recognizes the superior achievements of engineers. Dr. William A. Wulf is president of the National Academy of Engineering.

The **Institute of Medicine** was established in 1970 by the National Academy of Sciences to secure the services of eminent members of appropriate professions in the examination of policy matters pertaining to the health of the public. The Institute acts under the responsibility given to the National Academy of Sciences by its congressional charter to be an adviser to the federal government and, upon its own initiative, to identify issues of medical care, research, and education. Dr. Kenneth I. Shine is president of the Institute of Medicine.

The **National Research Council** was organized by the National Academy of Sciences in 1916 to associate the broad community of science and technology with the Academy's purposes of furthering knowledge and advising the federal government. Functioning in accordance with general policies determined by the Academy, the Council has become the principal operating agency of both the National Academy of Sciences and the National Academy of Engineering in providing services to the government, the public, and the scientific and engineering communities. The Council is administered jointly by both Academies and the Institute of Medicine. Dr. Bruce M. Alberts and Dr. William A. Wulf are chairman and vice chairman, respectively, of the National Research Council.

v

Consultants

ANDREA FISHMAN, Research Assistant, The Lewin Group, Falls Church, Virginia

DARRELL J. GASKIN, Research Assistant Professor, Institute for Health Care Research and Policy, Georgetown University Medical Center

JUDITH KRAUSS, Professor, Yale University School of Nursing

THOMAS C. RICKETTS III, Director, North Carolina Rural Health Research Program, Cecil G. Sheps Center for Health Services Research, and Associate Professor, Department of Health Policy and Administration, School of Public Health, University of North Carolina at Chapel Hill

LESLIE SCALLET, Vice President, The Lewin Group, Falls Church, Virginia

ANDY SCHNEIDER, Principal, Health Policy Group, Washington, D.C.

ALEXANDRA SHIELDS, Senior Research Associate, Institute for Health Care Research and Policy, Georgetown University Medical Center

REBECCA T. SLIFKIN, Senior Research Fellow, Cecil G. Sheps Center for Health Services Research, University of North Carolina at Chapel Hill

MICHAEL SPIVEY, Principal, Health Policy Group, Washington, D.C.

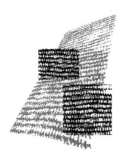 Preface

At a time of unprecedented prosperity and budget surpluses it seems almost out of style to focus on groups in our nation who fall outside the economic and medical mainstreams. These people include not only this country's 44 million uninsured individuals but also an almost equal number of low-income underinsured individuals. Vulnerable populations extend as well to poor and disadvantaged individuals living in inner cities and isolated rural communities, minority and immigrant families, people with special health care needs, and low-income groups who face a variety of other financial and nonfinancial barriers to stable health care coverage.

To address at least the basic health care needs of these impoverished and disadvantaged populations, America has long relied on an institutional safety net system, a patchwork of hospitals, clinics, financing, and programs that vary dramatically across the country. The funding and organization of the safety net have always been tenuous and subject to the changing tides of politics, available resources, and public policies. Despite their precarious and unstable infrastructure, these providers have proven to be resilient, resourceful, and adept at gaining support through the political process. Today, however, a more competitive health care marketplace and other forces of change are posing new and unprecedented challenges to the long-term sustainability of safety net systems and hold the potential of having a serious negative impact on populations that most depend on them for their care.

Our committee was asked to examine the impact of Medicaid managed care and other changes in health care coverage on the future integrity and viability of safety net providers, particularly core safety net providers such as community health centers, public hospitals, and local health departments. To carry out its charge, the committee reviewed the evidence from the peer-reviewed literature, held a 2-day public hearing, and elicited a broad array of expert testimony. The committee also conducted a number of regional meetings and commissioned several papers to provide further analyses on topics of special relevance to the study charge. In the course of our work, we were impressed by a number of excellent ongoing studies and surveys under way to determine how safety net providers and vulnerable populations are faring in the new environment. Much of this work is being sponsored by major health care foundations. At the same time, the committee was struck by the dearth of reliable and consistent data that can be used to accurately assess, measure, or compare the changing status of safety net systems across the country. Compounding the difficulty of accurate measurement is the ongoing evolution of Medicaid managed care and the turbulent health care environment.

These limitations notwithstanding, the committee came away from its deliberations convinced that today's changing health care marketplace is placing core safety net providers in many communities at risk of not being able to continue their mission of caring for a growing number of uninsured at a time when other national, federal, state, and local initiatives to expand coverage are still on the drawing board, in a fledgling state, or falling short of their promise. The growth of Medicaid managed care enrollment, the retrenchment or elimination of key direct and indirect subsidies that providers have relied upon to help finance uncompensated care, and growing demand for charity care are making it more difficult for many safety net providers to survive. Moreover, in many communities these adverse forces are affecting safety net providers all at once, placing already fragile underpinnings in even greater danger of falling apart.

In the absence of agreement on broader health care reform and with growing demand for charity care, the committee came to feel strongly that our nation's core safety net provider system needs to be sustained and protected. At the same time, the committee realized the importance of encouraging safety net providers to actively embrace the positive aspects of current change, including incentives to develop more integrated and accountable delivery systems and a greater emphasis on performance and customer service. Together with the committee's findings and recommendations, this report includes a synthesis of what the committee heard and learned over its 18 months of deliberations. We hope that our work will contribute in some small way to the dialogue on broadening the reach of access to health care for all Americans.

Stuart Altman, Ph.D.
Chair
March 2000

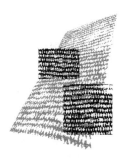

Acknowledgments

This volume has benefited from the encouragement, time, and expertise of many people. Efforts to accurately capture and document the status of America's health care safety net amidst the shifting sands of a tumultuous health care marketplace depended in important ways on generous help from a range of experts and knowledgeable colleagues. Although it is not possible to mention by name all of those who contributed to this study, the committee wants to express special appreciation to a number of groups and individuals for their valuable help.

Particular thanks are extended to the major sponsor of the study, the U.S. Department of Health and Human Services, Health Resources and Services Administration, and its administrator, Claude Earl Fox, M.D., M.P.H., for their support, patience, and thoughtful attention. We are especially indebted to Rhoda Abrams and Alex Ross for their enormous help. Before Alex came on board, Jennifer Friedenholtz contributed to the planning of the committee's public hearing. Marilyn Gaston, Michael Millman, and Jessica Townsend provided valuable early guidance and input. Special words of thanks go to Bonnie Lefkowitz for her unstinting generosity in helping the committee identify and analyze needed data. The contributions of Richard Bohrer, Wayne Meyers, and Robert Politzer were also greatly appreciated.

The committee also is greatly indebted to Medi-Cal Policy Institute in Oakland, California, and The Commonwealth Fund of New York for sponsoring regional meetings in California and New York, respectively, that helped the committee gain a firsthand understanding of the diversity of safety net organizations across the country. Valerie Lewis, Crystal Hayling, Brian Biles, and David Sandman deserve special praise for their help in developing these important meetings. Appreciation goes as well to James Tallon and the United Hospital Fund for hosting a meeting in the early stages of the study.

The committee wants to give special thanks to the dedicated and hardworking staff at the Institute of Medicine. We are particularly fortunate that Marion Ein Lewin agreed to take on the responsibilities of study director for the project. Marion brought to this effort a knowledge of the issues surrounding safety net providers and the individuals whose research activities and experience were most important for our evaluation. Above all, Marion's tireless energy, enthusiasm and commitment to excellence pushed the committee to produce what we believe is a first rate report. Judith Krauss, the 1998–1999 Institute of Medicine/American Academy of Nursing/American Nurse Foundation's Senior Nurse Scholar, contributed in major ways not only to the content of the report but also to many of the other lofty and mundane tasks that this kind of effort involves. Kari McFarlan deserves major commendation for her masterful and proficient handling of communications with the committee, organizing the literature database, and carrying out a myriad of other critical administrative tasks with great professional aplomb. Justine Lang deserves thanks for her administrative help in the early stages of this report and organizing the committee's first site visit to Tampa, Florida. Project assistant Michael Conroy was also helpful to the committee's work.

We thank Michael Hayes not only for his careful and professional editing but also for his interest in the project and thoughtful ongoing support. The committee also appreciated Richard Sorian's editing help from the perspective of his communications and health policy expertise. The committee owes countless thanks to Heather Binder, who "adopted" the study in its final months of gestation. Heather meticulously incorporated all of the edits and checked and double-checked all of the references, charts, and figures. Her proficient and careful review of the draft was a major contribution to the quality of the final product. Claudia Carl and Mike Edington provided assistance during the report review and preparation stages.

The committee wishes to express heartfelt appreciation to the authors of the commissioned papers. The well-researched and highly informative background papers enhanced the committee's understanding of the many dimensions of this complex issue. Alexandra Shields not only authored one of the commissioned papers but also conducted a national survey of local health departments with Magda Peck and contributed significantly to the research and writing of the report. Marlene Niefeld deserves thanks for her research assistance.

The committee extends special thanks to all of the people who contributed to the substance, learning, and enjoyment of our site visits. The committee is especially thankful to Bob Master, Jim Hooley, Jim Bernstein, Bill Remmes, Jane McCaleb, Patricia Bean, and Commissioner Thomas Scott for their help in planning and organizing these activities. The committee greatly appreciates the help and contributions of Christine Burch, Joel Cantor, Peter Cunningham, Lynn Fagnani, Marilyn Falik, Paul Fronstin, Darrel Gaskin, Brad Gray, Dan Hawkins, John Holohan, Robert Hurley, Lucy Johns, Ronda Kotelchuck, Leighton Ku, Debbie Lewis-Idema, Jack Needleman, Stephen Norton, and Sara Rosenbaum. These respected experts were never too busy to answer our calls, respond to our inquiries, and give generously of their time and knowledge. Thanks go as well to Joe Anderson, Jack Ashby, Amy Bernstein, Maura Bluestone, Dennis Braddock, Carol Brown, Bruce Bullen, Thomas Chapman, Lisa Tremento Chimento, Anne Dievler, Susanne Felt-Lisk, Irene Fraser, Marsha Gold, Eric Holzberg, Pat Jerominski, Neva Kaye, Peter Kralovec, Larry Lewin, Jack Meyer, John Murphy, Bill Sappenfeld, George Schieber, Bruce Siegel, Helen Smits, David Sundwall, Caroline Taplin, Pat Taylor, and Andrew Wallace for their thoughtful and informed perspectives.

Finally, the committee would like to thank the chair, Stuart Altman, for his intellectual leadership and for his strong commitment to the purposes of this project. He, in turn, wishes to thank the excellent and hardworking committee members whose dedication and perseverance to this effort far exceeded any reasonable expectations.

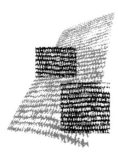 Reviewers

The report was reviewed by individuals chosen for their diverse perspectives and technical expertise in accordance with procedures approved by the National Research Council's Report Review Committee. The purpose of this independent review is to provide candid and critical comments to assist the authors and the Institute of Medicine in making the published report as sound as possible and to ensure that the report meets institutional standards for objectivity, evidence, and responsiveness to the study charge. The content of the review comments and the draft manuscript remain confidential to protect the integrity of the deliberative process. The committee wishes to thank the following individuals for their participation in the report review process:

GERARD F. ANDERSON, Director and Professor, Center for Hospital Finance and Management, Johns Hopkins University
JAMES BERNSTEIN, Director, North Carolina Office of Research, Demonstrations, and Rural Health Development, Raleigh
JO IVEY BOUFFORD, Dean, Robert F. Wagner Graduate School of Public Service, New York University
JAMES W. CURRAN, Dean and Professor of Epidemiology, The Rollins School of Public Health, Emory University
MARSHA R. GOLD, Senior Fellow, Mathematica Policy Research, Inc., Washington, D.C.

KEVIN GRUMBACH, Chief, Family and Community Medicine, San Francisco General Hospital/Community Health Network and Vice-Chair, Department of Family and Community Medicine, University of California at San Francisco

ROBERT HURLEY, Associate Professor, Department of Health Administration, Medical College of Virginia,Virginia Commonwealth University

RONDA KOTELCHUCK, Executive Director, Primary Care Development Corporation, New York City

JOSEPH P. NEWHOUSE, John D. MacArthur Professor of Health Policy and Management, Harvard University

MARK V. PAULY, Chair, Health Care Systems Department, The Wharton School of Finance, University of Pennsylvania

DAVID J. SANCHEZ, Jr., Commissioner, Health Commission, City and County of San Francisco

While the individuals listed above provided many constructive comments and suggestions, responsibility for the final content of the report rests solely with the authoring committee and the Institute of Medicine.

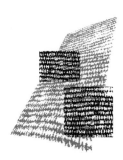

Contents

TABLES, FIGURES, AND BOXES

Figures

Tables

Boxes

America's
Health Care
SAFETY NET

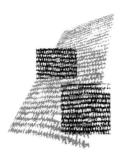 Executive Summary

Rising numbers of uninsured Americans, an increasingly price-driven health care marketplace, and rapid growth in enrollment of Medicaid beneficiaries in managed care plans may have critical implications for the future viability of America's health care safety net that serves a large portion of low-income and uninsured Americans. Of particular concern is the future of "core" safety net providers, institutions and physicians with a high level of demonstrated commitment to caring for uninsured and underserved patients. A failure to support and maintain these core providers could cause the entire safety net to collapse.

Despite the nation's vast riches and enormous resources, certain populations (referred to as "vulnerable populations" throughout this report) continue to fall outside the medical and economic mainstream and have little or no access to stable health care coverage. These populations include the 44 million Americans who are uninsured, low-income underinsured individuals, Medicaid beneficiaries, and patients with special health care needs who rely on safety net providers for their care. A large number of individuals who make up these groups are of minority and immigrant status and live in geographically or economically disadvantaged communities. The relationship between health insurance and access to health care and medical outcomes has been well documented (American College of Physicians-American Society of Internal Medicine, 2000; Davis and Schoen, 1977). Uninsured individuals are less likely to have a regular source of care, are more likely to report delay seeking care, and are more likely to report that they have not received needed care. Uninsured Americans may be up to three times more likely than privately insured individuals to experience adverse health outcomes and four times as likely as insured patients to require both avoidable hospitalizations and emergency hospital care (American College of Physicians-American Society of Internal Medicine, 2000).

In the absence of universal comprehensive coverage, the health care safety net has served as the default system for caring for many of the nation's uninsured and vulnerable populations. Until the nation addresses the underlying problems that make the health care safety net system necessary, it is essential that national, state, and local policy makers protect and perhaps enhance the ability of these institutions and providers to carry out their missions. In many communities these providers uniquely offer care that addresses the clinical and social needs of vulnerable patients who remain outside the economic and medical mainstream. Failure to support these essential providers could have a devastating impact not only on the populations who depend on them for care but also on other providers that rely on the safety net to care for patients whom they are unable or unwilling to serve.

To gain a better understanding of the potential impact of the current transformations in health care delivery, financing, and public policies on safety net providers, the U.S. Department of Health and Human Services' Health Resources and Services Administration asked the Institute of Medicine (IOM) to appoint a committee that would

> examine the impact of Medicaid managed care and other changes in health care coverage on the future integrity and viability of safety net providers operating primarily in ambulatory and primary care settings.

A committee of 14 experts was selected to conduct the study. The committee was carefully formulated to reflect a balance of expertise particularly relevant to its charge. The committee met five times between December 1997 and February 1999, and its deliberations and fact-finding activities included expert hearings and testimony, commissioned papers and data analyses, structured interviews, and site visits. These activities are described in greater detail in Chapter 1 of this report.

Although the committee understood that the study's sponsor was particularly interested in the ambulatory and primary care providers that fall under its funding authority, the committee and sponsor recognized that an accurate assessment of the role and future viability of these providers would have to encompass other major inpatient and community-based ambulatory care providers with demonstrated commitment to serving the poor and uninsured.

In carrying out its charge, the committee was asked to focus on the current challenges facing historical providers of care to the poor and uninsured in terms of their future financial viability and survival. In discussing its mandate, the committee was fully aware that this particular focus and perspective necessarily would exclude a broader exploration of alternative frameworks for providing the nation's poor and uninsured access to health care. In an environment of choice and competition, certain subgroups of traditionally safety net-dependent patients may have new and perhaps better care options. Some analysts argue that the future viability of safety net providers should be of concern only to the extent that these providers specifically and measurably improve access to quality health care for individuals in need of their services. Additionally, although traditional safety net providers serve a disproportionate number of poor and uninsured patients, in the aggregate they provide only a portion of the uncompensated care provided in most communities (Cunningham and Tu, 1997; Lefkowitz and Todd, 1999). This perspective could argue for a more global assessment of safety net services and their relative adequacy in a given community. Still others argue that policy and program efforts directed to poor and uninsured populations primarily should be targeted at broadening access to affordable insurance rather than subsidizing a designated class of providers.

Although the committee sees some merit in all of these perspectives, its charge was to assess the health care safety net system as it exists today and to focus its deliberations on these major providers of care to poor and uninsured populations. In addition, over the course of its deliberation the committee read and heard convincing evidence that even within the context of insurance reform segments of America's most disadvantaged populations will continue to rely on traditional safety net providers for their health care services, not only because these may be the only providers available and accessible, but also because many of these providers are uniquely organized and oriented to the special needs of low-income and uninsured populations.

Although no commonly accepted definition of the safety net exists, for the purposes of this study, the IOM committee defines the "health care safety net" as follows:

> Those providers that organize and deliver a significant level of health care and other related services to uninsured, Medicaid, and other vulnerable patients.

In most communities there is a subset of the safety net that the committee describes as "core safety net providers:"

> These providers have two distinguishing characteristics: (1) either by legal mandate or explicitly adopted mission they maintain an "open door," offering access to services for patients regardless of their ability

to pay; and (2) a substantial share of their patient mix is uninsured, Medicaid, and other vulnerable patients.

Core safety net providers typically include public hospital systems; federal, state, and locally supported community health centers (CHCs) or clinics (of which federally qualified health centers [FQHCs] are an important subset); and local health departments. In most communities several smaller special service providers (e.g., family planning clinics, school-based health programs, and Ryan White AIDS programs) also are considered a part of the core safety net. In some communities teaching and community hospitals, private physicians, and ambulatory care sites with demonstrated commitment to serving the poor and uninsured fulfill the role of core safety net providers.

The nation's health care safety net is not comprehensive, nor is it well integrated (Baxter and Mechanic, 1997). Rather, it is a patchwork of institutions, financing, and programs that vary dramatically across the country as a result of a broad range of economic, political, and structural factors. These factors include the strength and configuration of the local economy, the numbers and concentration of poor and uninsured individuals, the structure of the local tax base, the depth and breadth of a state's Medicaid eligibility and benefits, and the community's historic commitment to care for the uninsured and other vulnerable populations.

Although it is difficult to generalize about the overall state of the nation's health care safety net given its local nature and attributes, in carrying out its charge the committee was particularly concerned about the state of the core safety net and its ability to continue to provide needed access to this nation's most disadvantaged and underserved populations. In many underserved inner-city and rural communities, core safety net providers may be the only available source of primary health care services for the vulnerable populations residing in these areas.

Rising numbers of uninsured patients, coupled with changes in Medicaid policies and cutbacks in public and other subsidies, are beginning to place America's health care safety net in a state of serious jeopardy. The loss of safety net providers could harm not only the uninsured and people with low incomes but also the community at large. For example, in many regions, large public teaching hospitals are often the only source of trauma care, burn units, and other specialized services that are vital but that tend to be unprofitable.

THE THREAT TO CORE SAFETY NET PROVIDERS

Core safety net providers serve a disproportionate share of low-income and uninsured patients. In 1997, public hospitals provided 28 percent of their services to uninsured patients, and an additional 33 percent were to Medicaid patients (National Association of Public Hospitals and Health Systems, 1999). Similarly, more than 40 percent of patients who receive care from FQHCs are uninsured, whereas an additional 30 to 40 percent are Medicaid beneficiaries (Bureau of Primary Health Care, 1998).

Over the years, Medicaid (and to a lesser extent Medicare) has become the financial underpinning of the safety net. Historically, Medicaid has provided the majority of insured patients for most safety net providers and has subsidized a substantial portion of care for the uninsured through such programs as disproportionate share hospital (DSH) payments and cost-based reimbursement for FQHCs. State and local government grants also represent an important but variable source of revenues for most safety net providers.

A major cause for concern is the committee's finding that Medicaid as well as other revenues and subsidies that in the past have helped support care for uninsured and other vulnerable populations are becoming more restricted at the same time that the demand on the safety net is rising. The pressures on the safety net in many communities are the result of both intended and unintended consequences of the new health care marketplace and recently adopted public policies. Although the full impact of these dynamics is still unfolding, the committee has identified several troubling trends.

- **The number of uninsured people is growing.**

More than 44 million people, or 18 percent of the total nonelderly population, lack health care coverage, an increase of 11 million over the past decade. New studies forecast that, absent major reform, the ranks of the uninsured will continue to grow substantially over the foreseeable future (Custer and Ketsche, 1999). Rising insurance costs relative to family income, the impact of welfare reform, and other factors have contributed to these trends. As a result, both public hospitals and CHCs are seeing an increased number of uninsured patients.

- **The direct and indirect subsidies that have helped finance uncompensated care are eroding.**

The Balanced Budget Act of 1997 (BBA) reduced some of the major direct public subsidies that have helped finance health care for indigent populations, including significant cuts in Medicaid DSH payments and the phaseout over 5 years of cost-based reimbursement for FQHCs. The recently passed Balanced Budget Refinement Act of 1999 places a 2-year moratorium on the scheduled repeal and extends the phaseout from 2003 to 2005. The 1999 Act also calls for a study to determine how CHCs should be paid in subsequent years (National Association of Community Health Centers, 1999). The committee also read and heard evidence that in a number of states, state and local funds are also being cut or frozen, despite growing needs (Holahan et al., 1998; Norton and Lipson, 1998). With the decline and planned phaseout of federal subsidies, local revenues become increasingly important to the future viability of safety net providers.

In some communities a substantial proportion of care for the uninsured is delivered by private physicians and institutions that do not fall within the committee's definition of core safety net providers (Cunningham et al., 1999; Mann et al., 1997). Although these patients may represent only a small part of these providers' total practice or business, in aggregate these providers deliver a significant amount of charity care. Historically, these providers have been able to cover most of their uncompensated care costs by shifting the costs to other payers. Recent data indicate that physicians who derive a major share of their practice revenues from managed care are less willing or able to provide charity care (Bindman et al., 1998; Cunningham et al., 1999). This is placing even more pressure on an already strained safety net system.

- **The rapid growth of Medicaid managed care is having many adverse effects.**

A number of core safety net providers operating in mandatory Medicaid managed care environments are experiencing a decline in Medicaid revenues because of a reduction in the absolute numbers of Medicaid beneficiaries, the diversion of some Medicaid beneficiaries to other providers, and lower payments by Medicaid managed care plans (Lefkowitz and Todd, 1999). Competition for market share and downward pressure on prices by private payers have made Medicaid patients relatively more desirable to providers that in the past have not been willing to serve this population, shifting some Medicaid patients away from traditional providers. The committee heard extensive evidence that these factors are challenging the continuing ability of some safety net providers to balance the need to maintain a financial margin and pursue their mission of providing care to the uninsured.

In the past, safety net providers have served two major groups of poor patients: the uninsured and those on Medicaid. Over the years these two groups have become inexorably linked both because of the transient nature of Medicaid eligibility and because other providers could not or would not serve them. Although they were not originally intended to subsidize care for the uninsured, Medicaid revenues have helped core safety net providers defray some of the overhead and infrastructure costs, freeing limited grant funds and other revenues to be directed more to supporting care for the uninsured.

Under the traditional Medicaid program, beneficiaries were responsible for finding a willing provider to care for them. In many communities, Medicaid-participating providers were few and far between and safety net providers were the only source of care for the poor. Today, many states are offering Medicaid beneficiaries the opportunity to enroll in private managed care plans with the promise of more choice of providers and facilities. Enhanced choice of quality providers is desirable as a matter of equity and can create incentives for all providers to improve their performance. At the same time, however, the shift of Medicaid patients away from safety net providers combined with the growing number of uninsured people may have the effect of destabilizing an already fragile safety net.

The categorical and episodic nature of Medicaid eligibility means that individuals tend to cycle on and off insurance, often with long spells of no insurance. Under the traditional Medicaid program, low-income individuals and families who lost Medicaid coverage would continue to see safety net providers without much interruption. Private managed care organizations have no legal responsibility or mission to continue to support the care of patients when they become uninsured. The committee is concerned that these new trends not only undermine the financial viability of core safety net providers but also impair the continuity of care for these patients.

Although managed care has been shown to improve access to primary care in some communities, Medicaid managed care appears to have major differences from commercial managed care. Compared with privately insured persons, Medicaid beneficiaries tend to be far more vulnerable, their needs more diverse, and their experience with and capacity for exercising choice more limited. They may also lack the resources to go "out of plan" if they are dissatisfied with their care. In addition, nonmedical services of special importance to vulnerable populations (e.g., enabling services such as translation services, transportation to clinic visits, and the provision of child care services, and outreach) may not be part of a managed care contract or amenable to a managed care infrastructure. Procedures that facilitate ease of beneficiary enrollment and the exercise of choice, together with adequate oversight of plan performance, take on special importance for this population. Unfortunately, many of these efforts are in a fledgling stage and vary widely from state to state.

During the course of its deliberations, the committee was struck by the complexity and variations of local safety net systems, their various dynamics and financial circumstances, and the lack of sufficient and comparable data that can be used to reach with confidence empirical conclusions in certain areas in this period of ongoing evolution. These observations were reinforced by a number of articles, evaluations, and research papers that highlighted the promise and problems of Medicaid managed care in a more competitive, performance-based environment. In most cases, these studies concluded that the promise has not yet been fully realized and that the problems, although worrisome, have not yet reached crisis proportions.

In summary, the committee finds that core safety net providers in most communities are experiencing the adverse effects of many forces. The safety net has historically functioned in a precarious environment, surviving through many shifts in the economy, in policy, and in funding. Today, however, the convergence of new and powerful dynamics—the growth of mandated Medicaid managed care, the retrenchment or elimination of key direct and indirect subsidies that help finance charity care, and the growth in the number of uninsured Americans—is beginning to place unprecedented strain on the health care safety net in parts of the country. These dynamics and their potential impact on access to care for the nation's uninsured and most disadvantaged populations call for more concerted public policy attention and concrete action. In light of these considerations, the committee offers the following findings and recommendations (described in greater detail in Chapter 7 of this report):

MAJOR FINDINGS

Finding 1. The shift to Medicaid managed care can have adverse effects on core safety net providers and the uninsured and other vulnerable populations who rely on them for care. These dynamics demand greater attention and scrutiny by policy leaders and administrative agencies at the federal, state, and local levels.

Finding 2. Managed care principles offer significant potential for improved health care for Medicaid patients, but implementation problems can undermine this potential.

Finding 3. The financial viability of core safety net providers is even more at risk today than in the past because of the combined effects of three major dynamics: (1) the rising number of uninsured individuals; (2) the full impact of mandated Medicaid managed care in a more competitive health care marketplace; and (3) the erosion and uncertainty of major direct and indirect subsidies that have helped support safety net functions.

Finding 4. The patchwork organization and the patchwork funding of the safety net vary widely from community to community, and the availability of care for the uninsured and other vulnerable populations increasingly depends on where they live.

Finding 5. The committee found that most safety net providers have thus far been able to adapt to the changing environment. Even for these providers, however, the stresses of these changes have made it increasingly difficult for them to maintain their missions while protecting their financial margins. In addition, the full consequences of changing market forces, increases in the number of uninsured, and reduced levels of reimbursement have not yet been felt by these providers in some communities. The committee further observed that the current capacity for monitoring the status of safety net providers is inadequate for providing timely and systematic evidence about the effects of these forces.

RECOMMENDATIONS

Recommendation 1. Federal and state policy makers should explicitly take into account and address the full impact (both intended and unintended) of changes in Medicaid policies on the viability of safety net providers and the populations they serve.

In making this recommendation, the committee believes that the following issues need heightened public policy attention:

• failure to take into consideration the impact on safety net providers of changes in Medicaid policy could have a significant negative effect on the ability of these providers to continue their mission to serve the uninsured population, particularly those who move back and forth between being eligible for Medicaid and being uninsured;
• the adequacy and fairness of Medicaid managed care rates;
• the erosion of the Medicaid patient base and the financial stability of core safety net providers that must continue to care for the uninsured population;
• the declining ability or willingness of non-core safety net providers to provide care for the uninsured population; and
• the current instability of the Medicaid managed care market including the rapid entry and exit of plans and the impact of this churning of program beneficiaries.

Recommendation 2. All federal programs and policies targeted to support the safety net and the populations it serves should be reviewed for their effectiveness in meeting the needs of the uninsured.

Major new forces have altered the financing and delivery of health care services, including the move to managed care by both private and public payers, the separation of care for Medicaid patients from care for uninsured individuals, the erosion and retrenchment of direct and indirect subsidies that have helped provide care for those without coverage, and the increasing concentration of care for the uninsured population among fewer providers. These dynamics call for a careful review of programs and policies that were designed to improve access to care for vulnerable populations and support the providers that serve them to make sure that that these programs are still effectively targeted to meet their original objectives. The committee believes that such an analysis is especially important given the growing number of uninsured Americans and the declining ability to meet their health care needs. Federal health care programs that provide direct or indirect support for safety net providers and for services for vulnerable populations should be reviewed and modified to ensure that any funding allocation formula specifies explicit criteria for the delivery of services to the uninsured population as a basis for support. Eligibility for Medicaid and Medicare DSH funds should also be reexamined to include a greater focus on the level and share of services for the uninsured. Although the committee believes strongly that no funds should be diverted from the core safety net, any funds that become available as a result of this reexamination should be distributed in a manner that ensures that providers of both ambulatory and inpatient care are eligible to receive support.

Recommendation 3. The committee recommends that concerted efforts be directed to improving this nation's capacity and ability to monitor the changing structure, capacity, and financial stability of the safety net to meet the health care needs of the uninsured and other vulnerable populations.

The committee believes that the fragility of local safety nets has the potential to become a national crisis, and therefore, it calls for stronger federal tracking, direction, and targeted direct support. At this time, no single entity in the federal government has the responsibility for monitoring and tracking the status of America's health care safety net and its ability to meet the needs of those who rely on its services. Various agencies have responsibility for programs and policies that affect one part of the safety net delivery system (e.g., the Health Resources and Services Administration, the Centers for Disease Control and Prevention, the Substance Abuse and Mental Health Services Administration, the Health Care Financing Administration, the Head Start program, the Indian Health Service, and the Departments of Veterans Affairs, Defense, Agriculture, and Housing and Urban Development), but no comprehensive, coordinated tracking and reporting capability exists. Although it acknowledges the appropriate roles and responsibilities of the various agencies and the benefits of state and local innovations, the committee believes that such a tracking capability could promote public accountability, as well as a more coordinated approach to data collection, technical assistance, and the application and dissemination of best practices.

A number of organizational settings could be considered for the placement of an enhanced safety net tracking and monitoring activity, including an existing agency, department, or program, or a newly established entity. Although the committee elected not to come to a final decision on where such an entity could be placed, it did discuss and identify the major organizational attributes that would be needed to enable a safety net oversight entity to successfully carry out its mission. The committee strongly believes that such an entity should be independent; organized as an ongoing activity with dedicated staff; nonpartisan in its membership; and include a range of expertise required to carry out its charge. Such an oversight body would affect a number of state and local entities and would cut across several federal agencies. In identifying these attributes the committee viewed with favor an organization like the Medical Payment Advisory Commission (MedPAC) with its mandate to report directly to Congress. Alternatively, the oversight body could reside in the executive branch at a Departmental level. As an example of the executive branch model, the committee was impressed with the work and impact of the President's Advisory Commission on Consumer Protection and Quality in the Health Care Industry. However, the Quality Commission had a limited term, consistent with its mandate to produce recommendations for action and implementation by other parts of the federal government and the private sector. The committee's proposed tracking and monitoring activity would require an ongoing term of operation, since its major function would be to assess, monitor, and report on the status of America's health care safety net over time. The committee in its deliberations referred to the monitoring and oversight entity as the Safety Net Organizations and Patient Advisory Commission (SNOPAC).

To carry out its mission, the committee recommends that the initial activities of a safety net oversight entity include the following:

- monitor the major safety net funding programs (e.g., Medicaid, the

State Children's Health Insurance Program [SCHIP], Title V, FQHCs, and the various government DSH payment plans) to document and analyze the effects of changes in these programs on the safety net and the health of vulnerable populations;

• track the impact of the BBA of 1997 and other forces on the capacity of other key providers in the safety net system to continue their supportive roles in the core safety net system;

• monitor existing data sets to assess the status of the safety net and health outcomes for vulnerable populations;

• wherever possible, link and integrate the existing data systems to enhance their current ability and to track changes in the status of the safety net and health outcomes for vulnerable populations;

• support the development of new data systems where existing data are insufficient or inadequate;

• establish an early-warning system to identify impending failures of safety net systems and providers;

• provide accurate and timely information to federal, state, and local policy makers on the factors that led to the failures and the projected consequences of such failures;

• help monitor the transition of the population receiving Supplemental Security Income into Medicaid managed care including careful review of the degree to which safety net-based health plans have the capacity (e.g., case management and management information system infrastructure) to provide quality managed care services to this population and the degree to which these plans may be overburdened by adverse selection; and

• identify and disseminate best practices for more effective application of the lessons that have been learned.

> **Recommendation 4. Given the growing number of uninsured people, the adverse effects of Medicaid managed care on safety net provider revenues, and the absence of concerted public policies directed at increasing the rate of insurance coverage, the committee believes that a new targeted federal initiative should be established to help support core safety net providers that care for a disproportionate number of uninsured and other vulnerable people.**

Funding would be in the form of competitive three-year grants. Grants will vary in size, based on the scope of the project. Sources of financing could include funds available from the federal budget surplus and unspent funds from SCHIP and other insurance expansion programs. Although the committee projects such a new initiative may require a minimum of

$2.5 billion ranging over five years, the specific size and scope of this program should be determined by the administration and the U.S. Congress and should be modified based on an assessment of the parameters of the problem by the safety net oversight entity. These assessments should be an ongoing responsibility of the safety net oversight entity.

The following principles should govern the distribution of these funds:

- Because the committee recognizes the challenges of delivering coordinated, seamless care for the poor uninsured and other vulnerable individuals at a time when the number of such people is increasing, the new initiative should concentrate on both the infrastructure for such care and subsidies of the care itself. Multiple models could be funded under this initiative, mirroring the multiple models of safety net arrangements in the various states and local communities. For example, in some areas a large safety net hospital could take the lead and join with other providers, including community-based clinics. A state or local government could stimulate cooperative efforts in other areas, participating with its own service-delivery capacity. In still others, coalitions of ambulatory care providers, such as CHCs allied with local private physicians, could form and undertake the initiative.

- Funds could be used for infrastructure improvements (e.g., for equipment, rehabilitation of unattractive and inefficient buildings, and management information systems) or to help defray costs or support items and activities such as legal and other costs related to establishment of the network (in ways to avoid charges of antitrust and fraud and abuse), improvements in quality of care (e.g., patient tracking systems, re-engineering, and programs targeted to high-risk patients), and, where needed, the health care itself.

- Funds would be available to communities that demonstrate the potential capacity to deliver comprehensive services, to track patients and their outcomes as they move through the system, and to provide appropriate outreach and marketing efforts to reach patients with special needs. The allocations would specifically reward initiatives with demonstrated commitment and capacity to improve access and health outcomes for poor uninsured individuals in the community. Continuation of funding would be based upon ongoing satisfactory performance and accountability.

- Eligibility for funding would include a maintenance of effort requirement with documentation that the new funding would supplement and not replace state or local funding already directed to this effort.

During the time the committee was completing its study, the U.S. Department of Health and Human Services (DHHS), as part of its FY 2000 budget request, proposed a five year initiative designed to increase the capacity and effectiveness of the nation's health care safety net providers. To begin this effort, $25 million in the form of grant funding was appropriated under the FY 2000 Appropriations Act. The committee believes this new national program, the Community Access Program, which will provide funding for approximately 20 communities in the coming year, represents a good first step.

> **Recommendation 5. The committee recommends that technical assistance programs and policies targeted to improving the operations and competitive position of safety net providers be enhanced and better coordinated.**

Several federal agencies including the Health Resources and Services Administration, the Health Care Financing Administration, the Substance Abuse and Mental Health Services Administration, and the Centers for Disease Control and Prevention currently provide technical assistance to some safety net providers, but these funds are usually targeted exclusively to the programs and organizations funded by the respective agencies. The committee strongly believes that technical assistance funds should promote capacity building and the management and operating capabilities of all core safety net providers seeking to compete in a managed care environment. Technical assistance programs should promote rather than deter the development of partnerships and collaborations that can contribute to these objectives.

The committee believes the following areas require specific attention:

• management of service delivery and implementation of changes, including improvements in management information systems, appointment scheduling systems, patient telephone access, efforts to streamline operations, and reengineering of services so that they are more responsive to patients;

• development of new business skills such as negotiating managed care contracts and developing marketing techniques to maintain and expand the patient base of safety net providers;

• development and collection of reliable data on which to calibrate rates and assign appropriate risks to develop appropriate reimbursement systems; and

• nonmedical factors that affect utilization and health outcomes of low-income and other vulnerable patients using the health care delivery system (e.g., care-seeking behavior, cultural competence, and public health interventions).

CONCLUSIONS

The committee concludes that the safety net system is a distinct delivery system, however imperfect, that addresses the needs of the nation's most vulnerable populations. In the absence of universal insurance coverage and while the new market paradigms are unfolding, it seems likely that the nation will continue to rely on safety net providers to care for its most vulnerable and disadvantaged populations.

REFERENCES

American College of Physicians-American Society of Internal Medicine. 2000. *No Health Insurance? It's Enough to Make You Sick.* Philadelphia, PA: American College of Physicians-American Society of Internal Medicine.

Baxter, R., and Mechanic, R. E. 1997. The Status of Local Health Care Safety Nets. *Health Affairs, 16*(4), 7–23.

Bindman, A., Grumbach, K., Vranizan, K., Jaffe, D., and Osmond, D. 1998. Selection and Exclusion of Primary Care Physicians by Managed Care Organizations. *JAMA, 279*(9), 675–679.

Bureau of Primary Health Care. 1998. Uniform Data System. Bethesda, MD: Bureau of Primary Health Care/Health Resources and Services Administration, U.S. Department of Health and Human Services.

Cunningham, P., and Tu, H. 1997. A Changing Picture of Uncompensated Care. *Health Affairs, 16*(4), 167–175.

Cunningham, P., Grossman, J., St. Peter, R., and Lesser, C. 1999. Managed Care and Physicians' Provision of Charity Care. *JAMA, 281*(12), 1087–1092.

Custer, W., and Ketsche, P. 1999. *Health Insurance Coverage and the Uninsured: 1990–1998.* Washington, DC: Health Insurance Association of America.

Davis, K. and Schoen, C. 1977. *Health and the War on Poverty: A Ten-Year Appraisal.* Washington, DC: The Brookings Institution.

Holahan, J., Zuckerman, S., Evans, A., and Rangarajan, S. 1998. Medicaid Managed Care in Thirteen States. *Health Affairs, 17*(3), 43–63.

Lefkowitz, B., and Todd, J. 1999. An Overview: Health Centers at the Crossroads. *Journal of Ambulatory Care Management, 22*(4), 1–12.

Mann, J., Melnick, G., Bamezai, A., and Zwanziger, J. 1997. A Profile of Uncompensated Hospital Care, 1983–1995. *Health Affairs, 16*(4), 223–232.

National Association of Community Health Centers. 1999. *Compromise Delays Phase-Out of Health Center Payment System—Orders Congressional Report on Impact and Alternative Payment Mechanisms.* [WWW document]. URL http://www.nachc.com/FSA/Federal/Agenda/PPS/Compromise%20Announcement.htm (accessed February 1, 2000).

National Association of Public Hospitals and Health Systems. 1999. *America's Safety Net Hospitals and Health Systems.* Washington, DC: National Association of Public Hospitals and Health Systems.

Norton, S., and Lipson, D. 1998. *Portraits of the Safety Net: Public Policy, Market Forces, and the Viability of Safety Net Providers.* Occasional Paper No. 13. Washington, DC: The Urban Institute.

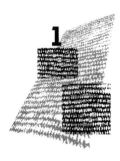

Background and Overview

BACKGROUND

A more competitive health care marketplace, changing federal policies, devolution of more responsibility to state and local governments, and the move to managed care have produced major changes in the financing and delivery of health care. An increasingly price-competitive environment has placed a greater premium on market share and has given hospitals and other providers strong incentives to merge and consolidate. Fee-for-service insurance is rapidly being replaced by systems of prepayment and risk-based capitation. There has been explosive growth in enrollment in managed care organizations. Between 1984 and 1993, the proportion of employees enrolled in health maintenance organizations (HMOs) increased from 5 to 50 percent. By 1998, 85 percent of employees with health insurance coverage were enrolled in some form of managed care (Kuttner, 1999). Ongoing pressures from government and private purchasers to make the system more cost-effective and efficient have shown some success. In 1997 health care spending rose a mere 4.8 percent, the slowest increase in nearly 40 years (Employee Benefit Research Institute, 1999).

The move to a new business paradigm for health care has unfolded against an increasingly troubling background—a rising number of uninsured Americans. In 1987, 31.8 million nonelderly Americans were uninsured. By 1998 this number had risen to 43.9 million, a 38 percent increase (Fronstin, 2000). In 1998, 18.4 percent of the total nonelderly population lacked insurance.

Growth in the ranks of the uninsured is occurring at a time when many of the major direct and indirect subsidies that have been critical to the financing of care for poor and uninsured patients are being restricted or are scheduled to be phased out. Although the care for these patients varies widely from state to state and even from community to community, responsibility for that care has in the past been shared by a broad array of hospitals, providers in outpatient care settings, and private physicians. In many communities a disproportionate share of the responsibility, however, has traditionally been sustained by a subset of public hospitals, teaching hospitals, community-based clinics, local health departments, and a discrete number of other institutions. Collectively, these organizations are known as the "health care safety net." Although the demand for free or discounted care is rising, the ability of the safety net to respond to the growing numbers of uninsured individuals is showing signs of deepening stress and some erosion (Kalkines, Arky, Zall and Bernstein, LLP, 1998; Baxter and Feldman, 1999). The increasing demands on safety net providers are being propelled in part by a reduction in the level of uncompensated care previously provided by non-safety net institutions and private practitioners (Cunningham et al., 1999; Mann et al., 1995).

America's health care safety net is a patchwork of providers, funding, and programs tenuously held together by the power of demonstrated need, community support, and political acumen. The safety net has never been particularly safe or secure, but changes in the current health care system in combination with rising numbers of uninsured may be placing the nation's health care safety net at a new level of risk.

In light of these trends, the U.S. Department of Health and Human Service's (DHHS's) Health Resources and Services Administration (HRSA) asked the Institute of Medicine (IOM) to undertake an 18-month study to:

> examine the impact of Medicaid managed care and other changes in health care coverage on the future integrity and viability of safety net providers operating primarily in ambulatory and primary care settings.

To conduct the study, a committee of 14 experts was selected and carefully formulated to reflect a balance of expertise particularly relevant to its charge.[1] The committee met six times between December 1997 and April 1999; its deliberations and fact-finding activities included site visits, regional meetings, structured interviews, and commissioned papers.

---

[1]Biographical sketches of the committee can be found in Appendix A.

APPROACH TO THE STUDY

Five tasks framed the committee's charge:

- First, to review and synthesize the evidence-based, peer-reviewed literature as well as other relevant articles and publications as they pertain to the major areas of the committee's scrutiny;
- Second, to guide, develop, and convene an expert hearing and workshop to highlight the leading research, policy, and model programs in this arena to assess what is known (or not known) about the current and projected status of safety net providers and the populations they serve;
- Third, to conduct two to three regional site visits to learn firsthand how various issues and policies related to the changing status of safety net providers are affecting the providers, administrators, and constituencies most directly involved in the day-to-day operations of safety net delivery systems;
- Fourth, to commission background papers on issues important to the committee that might not be adequately addressed in the expert hearing, workshop, and site visits; and
- Fifth, to produce a final report of the committee's findings, conclusions, and recommendations.

The committee conducted site visits and structured interviews in Tampa, Florida; Boston, Massachusetts; and rural North Carolina. During the course of the study, additional funding from the California Healthcare Foundation and The Commonwealth Fund made it possible for the committee to conduct two major regional meetings: in Oakland, California in December 1998, and in New York City in January 1999. The site visits and regional meetings helped inform the committee about important variations among states. These variations exist in both the organization and the strength of the safety net and in the adaptive strategies being developed to respond to Medicaid managed care.

The accumulated evidence from the literature, expert workshop, and regional site visits suggested four areas in need of more in-depth exploration: (1) special safety net issues for rural providers, (2) a better understanding of the parallel issues in behavioral health, (3) an analysis and lessons learned from the Medicaid DSH program, and (4) an assessment of data resources and information gaps. To gain more specific knowledge on these topics, the committee commissioned four background papers:

- The Changing Market, Managed Care and the Future Viability of

Safety Net Providers—Special Issues for Rural Providers, by T.C. Ricketts, R.T. Slifkin, and P. Silberman, 1998.
 • Behavioral Health Community Providers' Response to Managed Care, by G.K. Robinson, G.T. Bergman, S.E. Crow, and L.J. Scallet, 1998.
 • Issues in Designing a Fund for Safety Net Providers, by A. Schneider and M. Spivey, 1999.
 • Understanding the Role and Future Viability of Safety Net Providers: Data Resources and Information Gaps, by A.E. Shields.

The paper by Ricketts and colleagues was used as background for Chapter 2 on the structure and diversity of the safety net, and the one by Robinson and colleagues was used as background for Chapter 6 on special-needs populations. The third paper by Schneider and Spivey helped inform the committee's thinking about the design of future funding and policies targeted to helping providers who care for a disproportionate number of poor and uninsured patients. The fourth paper by Shields was used as background for Chapters 3 and for the committee to gain a better understanding of the special challenges associated with obtaining reliable, comparable, and timely data to assess and monitor the impact of the changing health care market on safety net providers.

In addition, the report includes two original figures developed by the committee:

 • Safety Net Providers: Keys to Successful Adaptation and Future Viability in a Managed Care Environment (Box 4.1, p. 155)
 • Characteristics of Medicaid Managed Care That Make It Different from Commercial Managed Care (Box 5.1, pp. 161–162).

With supplementary funding from HRSA, the committee was able to commission a number of analyses to address some important information gaps, including the following:

 • An analysis of national (American Hospital Association) hospital data (1991 to 1996) to ascertain whether greater price competition in the hospital market was leading to an increasing concentration of uncompensated care within the 100 largest metropolitan statistical areas at the same time as Medicaid revenues to these hospitals were declining. Reports from representatives of safety net hospitals at the committee's public hearing and site visits offered testimony indicating that the above phenomenon was taking place.
 • An independent analysis of the most recent (1997) Uniform Data System (UDS), the annual reports required by HRSA of all federally qualified health centers (FQHCs),[2] to assess changes in the patient and payer

mixes of these centers. During the later stages of the present study, 1998 UDS data became available for analysis and are discussed in Chapter 3 of this report.

• A national survey of local health departments to gain a better understanding of how they are responding to the new requirements of managed care.

ORGANIZATION OF THE REPORT

The report is divided into seven chapters:

• The remaining sections of Chapter 1 include a description of the committee's key definitions, study parameters, and caveats. In addition, for readers who may not have the time to read the report cover to cover, this chapter offers a summary of the major program and policy issues that form the context of this study. These issues are covered in greater detail in other chapters of this report.

• Chapter 2 includes an overview and brief history of the nation's major safety net systems, including their relative roles and importance, their patient and payer mixes, and their unique characteristics. This chapter also describes the chief structural characteristics of safety net systems.

• Chapter 3 provides the latest data on current forces affecting changes in the demand for, the support of, and the structures and environments of safety net systems. It also provides an assessment of the adequacy and gaps in current data systems.

• Chapter 4 reviews the data on how various safety net systems are responding to the changing market and what adaptive mechanisms are most critical to success.

• Chapter 5 reviews the literature on how the move to Medicaid managed care and other changes are affecting populations traditionally served by safety net systems.

• Chapter 6 examines the impact of Medicaid managed care on special-needs populations. Four groups (children with special needs, people with serious mental illness, people with HIV/AIDS, and people who are homeless) are used to highlight the literature and the experiences of the states in implementing Medicaid managed plans for these populations.

• Chapter 7 presents the committee's findings and recommendations.

---

[2]FQHCs qualify for Medicaid cost-based reimbursement and receive federal Section 330 grant funds under the Public Health Service Act. They include traditional community health centers, migrant health centers, Health Care for the Homeless Programs, and Public Housing Primary Care Programs (see Chapter 2).

KEY DEFINITIONS, STUDY PARAMETERS, AND CAVEATS

IOM Definition of Safety Net Providers and
Core Safety Net Providers

Even though the United States is a nation with vast riches and enormous wealth, it has failed to assure timely and effective access to health care for many populations. For some, the primary barrier is the lack of insurance. For other low income patients who may have insurance, there often remain serious barriers to care because of inadequate coverage, or non-financial impediments related to culture, education, transportation, language differences, homelessness, immigrant status, or difficult health problems (e.g., substance abuse, mental illness, HIV/AIDS). In this study, the IOM committee focuses on the health care problems of these "vulnerable populations" (i.e., uninsured individuals, underinsured individuals with low incomes, Medicaid recipients, individuals residing in medically underserved areas, and patients with special needs[3]) who are most at risk in our fragmented health care delivery system.

The institutions and professionals that by mandate or mission deliver a large amount of care to uninsured and other vulnerable populations are often referred to as "safety net providers." During its various deliberations, workshops, and site visits, the committee observed a general lack of agreement and ongoing debate on which providers constitute the health care safety net. In the absence of a universally accepted definition of the safety net, for the purposes of this study the IOM committee defines safety net providers as

> Those providers that organize and deliver a significant level of health care and other health-related services to uninsured, Medicaid, and other vulnerable patients.

In most communities, there is a subset of the safety net that the committee describes as "core safety net providers."

> These providers have two distinguishing characteristics: (1) by legal mandate or explicitly adopted mission they maintain an "open door," offering access to services to patients regardless of their ability to pay; and (2) a substantial share of their patient mix is uninsured, Medicaid, and other vulnerable patients.

By "substantial" the committee means providers who have a high

---

[3]Patients with special needs are people with serious chronic illnesses or disabilities as well as those who have experienced social dislocation (e.g., homelessness). Special needs populations are discussed in Chapter 6 of this report.

market share of uncompensated care and high commitment to such care as demonstrated by its ratio of uncompensated care to its total payer mix.

These core safety net providers typically include federal, state, and locally supported community health centers (CHCs) or clinics, public hospital systems, and local health departments. In some communities they also include mission-driven teaching hospitals, community hospitals, and ambulatory care clinics (which are often located in central city areas or which serve as the sole provider of health care in the community).

The committee discussed at length the desirability and feasibility of identifying a specific threshold or percentage of care to the uninsured that would have to be met before a clinic, hospital, or practitioner could be classified as a "core" safety net provider. During the course of its work, however, the committee was struck by the wide variations that exist across the country in (1) the demand for safety net services as measured primarily by the number of uninsured persons in a community, (2) the composition of the safety net and the concentration of care to the poor and uninsured, and (3) the market, political, and social environment in which local safety net providers operate. A review of the literature indicates that "there is no such things as an official health care safety net" (Rovner, 1996). An attempt to quantify safety net or disproportionate share providers for the purpose of Medicaid DSH funding has not guaranteed that funds are well targeted or allocated (Coughlin and Liska, 1998; Schneider and Spivey, 1999). Part of the problem has been the lack of accurate data on where uninsured people receive their care.

Given these findings and observations, the committee determined that it was inadvisable, if not impossible, to set a specific threshold that would be meaningful or relevant for all communities. There was a consensus that core safety net providers are those providers in a community whose disappearance would most hurt the poor and uninsured populations.

Some questioned whether Medicaid patients should be included in the committee's definition of "vulnerable populations," given their access to insurance coverage. The committee unanimously agreed to include Medicaid patients as "vulnerable" given historic concerns about payment rates to providers, the highly unstable and categorical nature of Medicaid coverage, the low socioeconomic status of Medicaid beneficiaries, and their often more complex health care needs. Moreover, the federal government identifies the uninsured and Medicaid beneficiaries as the two principal groups to be at high risk for medical underservice (Rosenbaum et al., 2000).

In defining "core safety net," the committee considered whether to limit its definition to only those providers who are *legally mandated* to care for uninsured patients and other vulnerable populations. Although this definition is often used, the committee, in its hearings and analysis of the data, came to recognize that in some communities, mission-driven hospitals, health care systems, clinics, and individual providers provide a substantial amount of such care, even though they are not legally mandated to serve these groups. For example, Detroit does not have a public hospital. The uninsured population in that city seeks inpatient and emergency room care primarily from Detroit Medical Center, a nonprofit academic medical center. In Milwaukee the public hospital (John Doyne) closed and the burden for taking care of the uninsured is shared among all hospitals. With the closing of John Doyne, a primary care delivery network was developed, anchored by a network of CHCs and clinics. These clinics act as gatekeepers for the provision of hospital care.

California gives counties significant discretion in determining their local safety net system. Los Angeles has built up a large public system of hospitals and clinics that, until recently, has not tried to partner with private providers in the county (Zuckerman et al., 1998). In contrast, San Diego County has no county-run hospitals or primary care clinics. Instead, the county contracts with private-sector, nonprofit groups to provide care for the indigent population. The county takes the role of catalyst rather than funder in the public-private collaboration (Zuckerman et al., 1998; California regional meeting testimony to the IOM committee, 1998).

In addition to New York City's Health and Hospital Corporation, the nation's largest public hospital system, 33 designated financially distressed and voluntary supplementary low-income patient adjustment (SLIPA) hospitals serve disproportionately large numbers of Medicaid and uninsured patients.[4] Although voluntary SLIPA and financially distressed hospitals represent less than one-fifth of the state's nonpublic hospitals, they account for 27 percent of all self-paying discharges and 48 percent of all Medicaid discharges delivered outside public hospitals (Kalkines, Arky, Zall and Bernstein, LLP, 1999).

The committee gives core safety net providers particular attention because they are likely to be more directly affected by increases in the number of uninsured, changes in Medicaid policies, and reductions in funding for programs that support care for poor and uninsured populations. Their narrow base of paying patients makes it difficult for these providers to shift expenses for uninsured patients to other payers. Moreover, their dependence on Medicaid revenues and federal, state, and local subsidies exposes these providers to exceptional financial risk if Medicaid payment levels are further reduced, if Medicaid patient volumes decline,

---

[4]Seventeen percent of New York State's residents lack coverage compared to a 50 state average of 15.6 percent. Almost one-half of New York City's population is either on Medicaid or uninsured.

or if other sources of direct or indirect support (e.g., disproportionate share hospital [DSH] payments and cost-based reimbursement for federally qualified health centers [FQHCs]) are reduced.

Traditionally, core safety net providers have served as the default health care system for poor and vulnerable populations. Even if universal health care coverage is someday realized, certain isolated and disadvantaged populations will continue to face significant barriers to care, including demographic, linguistic, cultural, racial, geographic, and organizational barriers (Darnell et al., 1995; Rosenbaum et al., 2000).

In many communities a substantial proportion of care for uninsured and vulnerable populations is provided by private physicians and institutions such as academic medical centers and not-for-profit hospitals not included in the committee's definition of the core safety net. In aggregate, these providers may deliver the majority of care for vulnerable populations in a community, and the committee recognizes their importance in assuring some level of access for many patients (Cunningham and Tu, 1997; Mann et al., 1997). These providers are not the focus of this report because the uncompensated care they provide to vulnerable populations represents a small share of their patient mix, and they have historically been able to absorb or cover these expenses by shifting the costs to other payers. However, given the growth of managed care, the increased competitiveness in the health care marketplace, and the pressures resulting from the Balanced Budget Act of 1997, the willingness and ability of many of these providers to continue their commitment to charity care may become impaired, placing even more pressure on a community's safety net (see Chapter 3).

The committee recognizes the complex dynamic that exists within a community among all of the providers that serve uninsured and other vulnerable populations. Visually, it may be helpful to picture this dynamic as several layers or "rings" around a central core. The relative size, patient care contribution, and organization of providers in each segment differs greatly from community to community. The current finite capacity, ability, or willingness of each ring or subset of providers to care for those with no or inadequate coverage makes this relationship strongly interdependent. The stability of the overall safety net is dependent on maintenance of effort of each of the segments, that is, if the core or the rings were to be significantly disrupted, the entire safety net would be in danger of coming apart. For example, without core safety net providers in many communities, other providers that serve the uninsured and other vulnerable patients may be unwilling or unable to assume the burden of caring for substantially larger numbers of patients. Conversely, the core safety net with its limited capacity and patchwork funding depends on the ongoing contribution of care to uninsured and other vulnerable patients made by the larger subsets of other community providers. This picture is further complicated by competition between providers in the core and rings for segments of the Medicaid population (e.g., healthy pregnant women) and, in some cases, for uninsured patients in communities where subsidies that support such care (e.g., uncompensated care pools and indigent care programs) are available.

Study Parameters and Caveats

The committee considered its work and statement of task at its first meeting in December 1997. As part of that discussion, the committee set some parameters and caveats regarding its work agenda.

Emphasis on Providers

In looking at the effects of the changing environment on the nation's health care safety net, the committee acknowledged that the ultimate goal must be to assess whether the needs of the communities and populations served by these providers are adequately met. However, these patients are served by providers, and in keeping with its charge, the committee focused its attention on the changing financial and organizational status of safety net providers, particularly core safety net providers. Nevertheless, the committee believes strongly that the future of these safety net providers in a more competitive marketplace will and should depend on whether the populations traditionally served by them will continue to choose these providers under conditions of enhanced choice. If over the long term, Medicaid patients become more attractive to the broader and more competitive health care market, safety net providers accustomed to a captive patient population may find themselves having to improve services or else lose their patient base and financial viability.

Community and Institutional Providers

Although the committee understood that the study's sponsor was particularly interested in community-based ambulatory care providers that fall under its funding authority, the committee and sponsor recognized that an accurate assessment of the role and future viability of these providers would have to include other important contributors to in- and outpatient care for vulnerable populations. These include public hospitals, local health departments, and clinicians working as a group or individually with demonstrated commitment to serving poor and uninsured populations.

Special-Needs Populations

The report devotes a chapter (Chapter 6) to the impact of Medicaid managed care on special-needs populations served by safety net providers. These populations are considered particularly medically and economically vulnerable and help highlight a number of the challenges in the expansion of Medicaid managed care beyond the Aid to Families with Dependent Children/Temporary Assistance to Needy Families population.

Expanded Choice of Providers

"Mainstreaming" (i.e., offering beneficiaries a choice of providers from beyond the core safety net) often is cited as a goal in extending managed care to vulnerable populations. The committee voiced concern that the concept of mainstreaming conveys certain values that may not reflect reality. Mainstream plans and providers may automatically be viewed as offering better care; that is, they are in the mainstream rather than at the margin or the periphery. During its fact-finding activities, the committee came to realize that Medicaid-dominated plans or safety net plans may be structured in ways that better meet the often complex health care needs and cultural diversity of vulnerable populations. In addition, Medicaid-dominated plans may be more likely to include providers that also serve the uninsured. Rather than the goal of mainstreaming per se, the committee believes that providing beneficiaries with improved opportunities for "informed choice of quality providers" may be a more important and meaningful objective.

Research Evidence and Empirical Observations

In carrying out its charge, the committee struggled with the limitations and lack of comparability of critical data for definitive assessment of the changing financial and organizational statuses of safety net providers and the populations they serve. The committee was asked to give its priority attention to primary care safety net providers operating in ambulatory care settings. Research and data collection activities have, however, focused primarily on hospitals and other institutional providers. In addition, survey data are available from relevant member organizations and advocacy groups[5] as well as HRSA, but these data are frequently limited

---

[5]American Hospital Association, National Association of Public Hospitals and Health Systems, National Association of Community Health Centers, and National Association of County and City Health Officials.

in a number of ways. For example, some surveys are not available for every year, because of resource and other constraints. Other surveys are fielded more regularly but address different content areas across years depending on the key policy and political priorities of special interest to the membership.

HRSA is the only national source of data for CHCs. The agency is required to collect annual data on the user and revenue profile of all FQHCs. Before 1995, however, data on users by payers were derived from grant applications rather than UDS reports, making longitudinal comparisons of users before and after 1995 unreliable. In addition, UDS data do not include CHCs that are not classified as FQHCs (Chapter 2 includes a discussion of the FQHC program).

The diversity of safety net organizations across the country and their ongoing evolution added to the committee's difficulty in collecting a reliable empirical evidence base for its findings and recommendations. State and local data vary widely in their availability, scope, quality, and timeliness.

Despite these limitations, the committee was able to review a substantial amount of peer-reviewed literature, timely case studies, and ongoing surveys and studies such as those being conducted by the Urban Institute, the Center for Studying Health System Change, the Henry J. Kaiser Family Foundation, the Commonwealth Fund, and Mathematica Policy Research, Inc.

The committee received additional timely information from site visits, a major public hearing conducted in Washington, D.C., expert testimony conducted throughout the course of the study, in-depth telephone interviews with leaders in the field, commissioned papers, and analyses conducted specifically for the report as described earlier in this chapter.

Alternative Views of the Safety Net

In carrying out its charge, the committee was asked to focus on the challenges to financial viability and survival facing traditional providers of care for poor and uninsured populations. In discussing its mandate, the committee was fully aware that this particular focus and perspective would necessarily exclude a broader exploration of alternative frameworks—such as universal coverage—for providing health care access to the nation's poor and uninsured. In an environment of choice and competition, patients may have new and perhaps better care options. Some analysts argue that the future viability of safety net providers should be of concern only to the extent that these providers specifically and measurably improve access to quality medical care for individuals in need of their services. Additionally, although core safety net providers serve a disproportionate number of poor and uninsured individuals, in the aggregate they provide only a portion of the uncompensated care provided in most communities. This perspective would argue that policy and program efforts targeted to the poor and uninsured should be focused on broadening access to affordable insurance rather than subsidizing a class of providers. Although the committee saw the merit of these perspectives, its charge was to assess the financial viability of the health care safety net system as it exists today and to focus its deliberations on the major providers of care to vulnerable populations. In addition, the committee also believed that although extending coverage is an important policy objective, no single incremental approach to restructuring and broadening the health insurance system is likely to address the diverse needs of the 44 million uninsured individuals in the United States. Given the limited resources this country has been willing to devote to health care for the uninsured, a safety net delivery system may be the most efficient and effective way to provide health care services to sizeable subsets of this population. Moreover, in many parts of the country, traditional safety net providers may be the only providers available and accessible to poor and uninsured populations.

Local Variations

The composition of the safety net and the concentration of responsibility for care for the poor vary dramatically across communities and are a function of the demand for such care (e.g., number of uninsured individuals), the depth and breadth of Medicaid coverage, the economic and political environment, as well as the level of state and local support for care for vulnerable populations (Norton and Lipson, 1998).

There also are distinct differences between urban and rural safety net structures (Ricketts et al., 1998). Although teaching hospitals and professional educational programs help support a significant amount of care for vulnerable populations in inner cities, these resources are not usually available in rural settings. Care for vulnerable populations in rural areas is delivered primarily through CHCs or clinics and is supplemented by the care delivered by private practitioners who may receive bonus payments, incentives, enhanced federal payments, or other forms of cross-subsidies.

A good understanding of the variations in the organization and financing of care for vulnerable populations across communities is necessary both to adequately address the question of whether the safety net is in trouble and to better fashion potential strategies for improvement (Baxter and Mechanic, 1997; Bovbjerg and Marsteller, 1998). The issue of differences in local capacity, demand, and commitment to the provision of care to vulnerable populations is receiving heightened attention, given the ongoing devolution of responsibilities in this area from the federal government to states and localities.

PROGRAM AND POLICY OVERVIEW

The Changing Medicaid Market

Evolution of Medicaid Managed Care

Following the success of large employers in at least temporarily slowing the growth in health care spending by moving workers to managed care, states have rapidly converted the traditional Medicaid fee-for-service system into a managed care program, using a range of risk-based and non-risk-based models. The move from the fee-for-service system to managed care has been fast and powerful. In 1998 managed care became Medicaid's dominant delivery system; more than half (16.7 million) of all beneficiaries are now enrolled in managed care (Kaye et al., 1999). Today, 48 states (all except Alaska and Wyoming) are pursuing some managed care initiatives. More than 75 percent of Medicaid beneficiaries in 10 states (e.g., Florida, Oregon, and Arizona) are enrolled in managed care (The Kaiser Commission on Medicaid and the Uninsured, 1998a).

States traditionally have moved to managed care to control their Medicaid costs, expand coverage for the uninsured, and make health care providers and plans more accountable for performance and quality (Horvath et al., 1997; Iglehart, 1995). In recent years, the political and policy environments in many states have produced a change in emphasis from the pursuit of coverage expansions to fiscal conservatism. As a result, the cost savings potential of Medicaid managed care has become the major lever driving program change (Henderson and Markus, 1996; Hurley and Wallin, 1998). Medicaid expenditures exploded between 1988 and 1992, mostly as a result of growth in enrollment attributable to an economic recession, a number of federal eligibility mandates, and the growth of DSH payments (Holahan and Liska, 1996).

Although Medicaid has increasingly been used to expand coverage to low-income groups, the program covers only half of Americans living below the poverty level. The categorical nature of Medicaid eligibility means that only persons with particular profiles such as low-income children, pregnant women, elderly people, and people with disabilities are eligible to enroll. Medicaid's restrictive rules and processes result in individuals cycling on and off eligibility on a regular basis. Only about one-third of all beneficiaries remain on Medicaid for more than a year; most of those who lose eligibility become uninsured (Carrasquillo et al., 1998).

According to the latest figures compiled by Health Care Financing Administration (HCFA), in 1997 Medicaid covered 41.3 million people at a cost of $160 billion.[6]

Although it is only in recent years that Medicaid managed care has been widely implemented, extension of the principles of managed care to low-income populations has had a longer and, at times, contentious history that has occurred in phases. The first phase was in the late-1960s, when the state of California sought to rapidly enroll its Medicaid (Medi-Cal) population in managed care plans as a way of controlling escalating expenditures. Low capitation rates kept many of California's mainstream plans and providers from entering this market. Entrepreneurs, hoping to capitalize on a new and potentially lucrative business, seized the opportunity to quickly develop a number of new plans that were understaffed, underqualified, and underfunded (Zuckerman et al., 1998). Fraudulent marketing and financial practices soon turned into scandals and became the subject of national headlines. These unfortunate developments and their negative impact on care for the poor in California raised early concerns in the U.S. Congress and elsewhere about the advisability of moving vulnerable populations into managed care and signaled the importance of instituting adequate regulations in this arena.

The passage of the Omnibus Budget Reconciliation Act (OBRA) of 1981 ushered in the second phase of Medicaid managed care development. The 1981 OBRA encouraged state-level experimentation with alternative forms of delivery of medical services. This second phase saw the creation of the nation's first statewide managed Medicaid program, Arizona's Health Care Cost Containment System, begun in October 1982. Up to that time, Arizona had been the only state that did not participate in Medicaid (McCall, 1996).

Despite growing interest on the part of states to use managed care as a vehicle to improve Medicaid provider participation and to stabilize program expenditures, the nationwide rate of enrollment in Medicaid managed care remained static at about 10 percent of Medicaid beneficiaries for most of the 1980s (Iglehart, 1995). On a voluntary basis Medicaid beneficiaries saw little advantage in giving up their freedom of choice of providers to enroll in a more restrictive delivery program. It was not until the passage of the Section 1915(b) freedom of choice and Section 1115 research and demonstration waivers that states gained the power to mandate managed care enrollment and to limit beneficiaries' freedom of choice.

---

[6]There is a 2-year delay in HCFA's publication of Medicaid enrollment data.

Section 1115 and 1915(b) Waivers

Named for the sections of the Social Security Act in which they are found, Section 1115 and 1915(b) [7] waivers fostered rapid expansion of mandatory Medicaid managed care. The Section 1115 waivers allow states to put aside almost any Medicaid requirement—from eligibility rules to payment requirements—subject to HCFA approval and the discretion of the Secretary of DHHS. So long as total program costs are budget neutral, any program savings can be used to expand coverage to other low-income people. The waivers also signified a shift in payment structure from direct payments to providers to direct payments to participating managed care entities. Safety net providers can in turn contract with these managed care entities, contract with the state Medicaid agency, or establish their own managed care plans (Lee, 1997).

The Section 1115 waivers contained special implications for FQHCs by eliminating the federal requirement established by the 1989 and 1990 OBRAs, which made these entities a unique set of Medicare and Medicaid providers, reimbursing them on the basis of "reasonable costs" for a defined set of services. Cost-based reimbursement ushered in an era in which FQHCs saw a significant growth in Medicaid users and revenues. Between 1990 and 1997, FQHCs increased their dependence on Medicaid, with revenues from Medicaid increasing from 21 to 35 percent of revenues (Lefkowitz and Todd, 1999).

Section 1915(b) waivers, in place in 40 states, are more limited but exempt states from federal rules concerning comparability and availability statewide, and permit them to implement mandatory managed care in part of the state or for certain categories of individuals (The Kaiser Commission on Medicaid and the Uninsured, 1998a). Section 1915(b) waivers also give states the right to allow plans to offer FQHC services without having to contract with FQHCs to provide those services (Rosenbaum and Darnell, 1997).

In most states, implementation of the waiver programs also expanded the willingness of other providers to participate in the Medicaid program because of changes in provider reimbursement. This has resulted in increased competition by providers for Medicaid patients.

Models of Medicaid Managed Care

States generally use two major Medicaid managed care models: risk-based plans and fee-for-service primary care case management (PCCM).

---

[7]Section 1115 waivers were originally introduced as part of the 1962 Public Welfare Amendments to the Social Security Act (P.L. 87–543) during the Kennedy Administration. Section 1915(b) waivers were part of the Medicaid Amendment promoted by Congress in 1981.

Under risk-based plans, a managed care organization (MCO) assumes financial risk for a defined set of health care services in exchange for a fixed payment per enrollee per month. Risk-based plans can be full-risk, in which an MCO assumes full-risk for the delivery of a comprehensive range of services, or partial-risk, in which an MCO contracts on a more limited basis (i.e., it provides only ambulatory care). In contrast, PCCM arrangements assign responsibility for the care of a Medicaid beneficiary to a specific primary care provider who receives payment on a fee-for-service basis and who (typically) receives a small additional fee per enrollee per month to compensate for case management functions.

As the market evolves and managed care becomes more pervasive, states are decreasing their reliance on PCCM arrangements and are moving toward risk-based plans (Holahan et al., 1998). As of June 1998, 585 Medicaid managed care plans, primarily full-risk HMOs, were in operation. This is double the number of such plans in 1993 (The Kaiser Commission on Medicaid and the Uninsured, 1999). There has been significant growth in the number of full-risk Medicaid plans, increasing from 196 in 1994 to 339 in 1997.

The vast majority (85 to 90 percent) of Medicaid enrollees in risk-based MCOs are children and women of child-bearing age (Holahan et al., 1998). Although this group makes up nearly three-fourths of beneficiaries, it accounts for only 27 percent of Medicaid spending. Given the predominance of low-cost beneficiaries currently enrolled in Medicaid managed care, overall program cost savings to states are projected to be small, in the range of 5 percent (Holahan et al., 1998). The potential of greater program savings will depend on whether managed care can be successfully implemented for the more costly low-income elderly and disabled populations, who have greater need for health care, with the accompanying high expenditures for that care.

Major Challenges of Medicaid Managed Care

Medicaid managed care may be fundamentally different from private sector managed care, requiring customization and special capabilities (Hurley and Wallin, 1998). From its inception in 1965, Medicaid's low reimbursement rates have limited provider participation, particularly in the area of primary care. Given the program's historically low payment rates, savings from managed care or the ability to negotiate with provider networks may be more difficult to realize. Compared with employed people, Medicaid beneficiaries have been shown to be much more vulnerable, their needs more diverse, and their experience with and capacity for exercising choice more limited. Because of their low-income status, Medicaid beneficiaries often lack the resources to "cost share" or to go "out of plan" if they are dissatisfied with their access to care.

The unstable eligibility of this group and short enrollment periods add to the complexity of providing care to this group. Although the move to broadened choice and managed care for Medicaid beneficiaries may well be a step in the right direction, contracts between Medicaid agencies and MCOs do not cover uninsured populations, nor do they provide for subsidies to furnish care for uninsured populations (Rosenbaum et al., 1998). Given the off-and-on nature of Medicaid eligibility, continuity of care for these patients, rather than being improved under managed care, may be at risk and disrupted if the plan cannot take care of beneficiaries when they lose coverage. In addition, contracts also do not typically cover services that are considered noncustomary within a commercial managed care contract, thereby leaving at risk some of the enabling and social support services so vital to maintaining and improving the health status of vulnerable populations.

Moreover, in addition to being an insurance program, Medicaid agencies have come to play multiple roles including protectors of state and local safety net systems, supporting a range of other community-based services together with medical education. Unlike commercial insurers, state Medicaid plans operate in a highly public and often politicized environment. Medicaid managed care has had to incorporate many of the program's unique roles, requirements, and limitations. Early experience indicates that survival of an MCO in the Medicaid market may require a commitment greater than that needed in other markets (Hurley and Wallin, 1998).

Pressures on the Safety Net

Growth in the Ranks of the Uninsured

As stated earlier in this report, despite a robust economy, almost 44 million nonelderly Americans lacked health insurance coverage in 1998. Even more disturbing are projections that if current trends continue, the uninsured population could balloon to nearly 47 million, or about 20 percent of the population, by 2005 (Thorpe, 1997). Most of the uninsured are low-income families (those with incomes of less than 200 percent of the federal poverty level), the target population that tends to rely most on core safety net providers for their health care.

Although the proportion of the population without insurance varies widely across states and regions, these variations are even more extreme among communities. For example, among the 12 communities being tracked by the Center for Studying Health System Change (CSHSC), the proportion of the population without insurance varies from 23 percent in Miami to 9 percent in Seattle (Cunningham and Pickreign, 1997). In the CSHSC tracking study the communities with large proportions of uninsured people also tend to have higher poverty rates and a much higher percentage of Hispanics. Labor market characteristics and the restrictiveness of eligibility for Medicaid and other public assistance programs are additional factors that explain the variations in rates of insurance coverage among states and communities.

In recent years some significant national efforts have been directed at incremental health reforms, but these programs are proving to have less than expected practical value for the growing numbers of uninsured Americans (Budetti, 1998). The Health Insurance Portability and Accountability Act of 1996 (also known as the Kassebaum-Kennedy law) was designed to make employer-provided group health insurance more portable between jobs and more available for employees who become self-employed or for individuals during periods of unemployment. Unfortunately, the premiums charged by many insurers for this expanded coverage have proved to be out of reach for most people with serious existing medical conditions.

Considerable hopes are being placed on the eventual success of the State Children's Health Insurance Program (SCHIP), a $24 billion 5 year program enacted as part of the Balanced Budget Act of 1997 (BBA) to help expand health insurance coverage to some of America's 11 million uninsured children. Under SCHIP, states may choose to expand Medicaid, to design or expand state-sponsored or private programs, or to use a combination of strategies to improve insurance coverage for uninsured, low-income children. Although the start-up of the program has been slower than expected, more than 1.3 million children were enrolled in the program at the end of June, 1999 (Alpha Center, 2000). Nevertheless, SCHIP enrollment to date has fallen considerably below original estimates, and one in seven children still lacks coverage (Perry et al., 2000). Lack of enrollment success has primarily been due to complex and burdensome enrollment procedures together with poor outreach efforts. Moreover, as the outlook for insurance coverage for children begins to show some signs of improvement, lack of coverage for millions of childless adults with low incomes and falling Medicaid rolls represent rising problems.

Several bills and policy proposals that will expand insurance coverage for low-income uninsured individuals are being discussed and debated in the 106th Congress. Most of these proposals are focused on using tax credits rather than mandates to reduce the nation's number of uninsured individuals. These proposals are part of a larger ongoing debate on the equity and perceived incentives of the current favorable tax treatment of employer-paid health insurance premiums extended to higher-income workers. A number of preliminary assessments of these proposals suggest although tax credits may improve equity in the financing of health insurance premiums, they probably are not an effective way to help low-income uninsured individuals gain coverage (Gruber and Levitt, 2000).

The Balanced Budget Act of 1997

The BBA of 1997 significantly revised and expanded the managed care policy options available to states under federal Medicaid statutes. The law grants states new authority to mandate managed care enrollment without obtaining a federal waiver (except for special-needs children, persons eligible for both Medicaid and Medicare, and Native Americans). The BBA of 1997 also waives a previous requirement that 25 percent of a plan's enrollment be privately insured (the 75/25 rule) and replaces it with a number of required managed care safeguards that states must build into their programs if they are to receive federal funding (Box 1.1). States with Section 1915(b) and 1115 waivers are exempt from these new requirements.

Of particular importance to FQHCs, the BBA of 1997 phases out cost-based reimbursement for FQHCs over 5 years.[8] Although the BBA Refinements Act of 1999 extends the year of final repeal from 2003 to 2005 and reduces the scope of the annual decreases in cost-based reimbursement between now and 2005, the eventual repeal of cost-based reimbursement is projected to have a significant impact on the ability of many FQHCs to maintain their mission of caring for rising numbers of uninsured individuals.[9]

During the transition, FQHCs are not to receive less for treating Medicaid enrollees in MCOs than for caring for beneficiaries under fee-for-service arrangements. States can opt to continue cost-based payments if they wish. At present approximately 27 states continue some type of cost-based reimbursement. However, public testimony to the committee underscored that such state support is, in most cases, fragile and temporary because it is highly dependent on the economy and because of competing demands for limited dollars.

---

[8]Before 1997, a number of states such as Oregon, Hawaii, Rhode Island, and Tennessee were allowed to waive FQHC coverage and payment rules as part of their Section 1115 demonstrations. Thus, some safety net providers were affected before the federal policy shift.

[9]Under the provisions of the BBA of 1997, the loss of cost-based reimbursement over five years was estimated to be as much as $1.1 billion; the 1999 BBA Refinements cuts these losses by approximately half (National Association of Community Health Centers, 1999).

**BOX 1.1 Medicaid Managed Care:
Selected Provisions in the Balanced Budget Act of 1997**

Enrollment/Marketing: Permits states to mandate managed care enrollment, guarantee enrollment for 6 months for adults and 12 months for children, and "lock in" beneficiaries for up to 1 year; door-to-door marketing is prohibited; and default enrollment systems must consider existing physician-patient relationships.

Plan Choice: Permits states to limit Medicaid beneficiaries to a choice of two MCOs in urban areas and one MCO in rural areas. Plans may serve Medicaid beneficiaries exclusively.

Access: Requires MCOs to comply with a "prudent layperson" emergency care standard and prohibits physician "gag rules."

Consumer Protections: Requires states to provide comparative information on MCOs including a list of participating plans, the benefits package and cost-sharing, out-of-plan covered benefits, service area, and quality and performance indicators. Other information, available if requested, includes the identity and location of providers, enrollee rights and responsibilities, and grievance and appeals procedures.

MCO Payment Rates: Requires that state Medicaid agency capitation payments be made on an "actuarially sound basis."

Plan Requirements: Requires plans to demonstrate adequate capacity, including an appropriate range of services and a sufficient number, mix, and geographic distribution of providers.

Quality/Oversight: Increases the threshold for prior federal approval of managed care contracts to $1 million, requires states to develop and implement a quality assessment and improvement strategy by 1999, and establishes external independent review of MCO performance.

SOURCE: The Kaiser Commission on Medicaid and the Uninsured (1998b). Reprinted with permission.

The BBA of 1997 also allows MCOs to provide the augmented services offered by FQHCs without specifically contracting with these providers. The BBA of 1997 generally leaves vague the terms of any contractual arrangements MCOs might elect to enter into with FQHCs (Alpha Center, 1998).

The BBA of 1997 contains a number of other provisions designed to achieve federal savings by reducing Medicaid reimbursements to hospitals generally and to "disproportionate share" hospitals in particular. The BBA of 1997 still requires states to make additional payments to hospitals that serve large numbers of Medicaid or uninsured patients, but it limits the federal Medicaid matching funds available for these DSH payments in each state.

Under the BBA of 1997, states that want to limit Medicaid beneficiaries living in urban areas to a choice between two MCOs can do so without seeking a waiver from the Secretary of DHHS. States can also limit beneficiaries living in rural areas to a single MCO. The Act contains provisions that help stabilize plan enrollment to address the cyclical nature of Medicaid eligibility. States are given the option to impose an annual lock-in with a 90-day open-enrollment period and can, if they choose, guarantee 6 months of Medicaid eligibility to any beneficiary or guarantee 12 months of eligibility to children up to age 19. A 1999 survey by the National Academy for State Health Policy indicates that a number of states are investing in continuity of care by increasing their use of lock-ins and guaranteed eligibility (Kaye et al., 1999).

The broader participation of core safety net providers in managed care was given a major boost by a provision in the BBA of 1997 that for the first time permits states to contract with Medicaid-only MCOs without first obtaining a federal waiver. Managed care plans sponsored by providers (called provider-sponsored organizations [PSOs]), such as CHCs or hospitals, can participate in Medicare and Medicaid independently of insurance companies. PSOs must be licensed under state law as risk-bearing entities, and the federal government must certify that they meet the requirements necessary to provide care to the Medicare population. Such plans must also adhere to federal consumer protections or to state protections if the latter are more stringent. PSOs can, however, obtain a waiver from state licensure that permits them to operate without the requirement of large reserves, taking into account their ability to provide services as assets against insolvency (National Association of Public Hospitals and Health Systems, 1997).

An analysis of the BBA of 1997 prepared for The Kaiser Commission on the Future of Medicaid concluded that the Act does not articulate a clear policy for the support of safety net providers in that it contains provisions that may both harm and benefit them (Schneider, 1997). Although some provisions of the BBA of 1997 reduce Medicaid reimbursements to safety net providers, other provisions make it easier for safety net providers to participate in managed care by liberalizing solvency requirements for this group. The analysis suggests that the changes for safety net providers brought about by the BBA of 1997 will probably take a few years to assess and will likely vary significantly from community to community and state to state.

Changing Medicaid Managed Care Market

As revenues are squeezed across the health care industry, providers and health plans that previously shunned the Medicaid market have geared up to compete for Medicaid patients. The years 1992 to 1996 saw a sharp growth in HMO participation in the Medicaid market, a growth that included all market segments and all forms of profit and ownership status (Felt-Lisk and Yang, 1997). Efforts to expand choice for Medicaid beneficiaries through commercial managed care plans have recently hit some snags. Since 1997, commercial plans exited the Medicaid market in much greater numbers than in previous years and entered new Medicaid market less frequently (Felt-Lisk, 1999).

In exiting the Medicaid market, plans cite low capitation rates, declining profitability, and financially burdensome administrative requirements imposed by states as major reasons for exiting the Medicaid managed care business (Hurley and McCue, 1998). Moreover, as states have moved from voluntary to mandatory Medicaid managed care programs, HMOs have seen their profitability decline (Hurley and McCue, 1998). After initially offering fairly generous rates to attract plans into the Medicaid market, many states have lowered their rates and demanded more in areas of contract specification. Contributing further to the Medicaid managed care market turnaround among commercial plans were declining profits in other lines of business and lower-than-expected Medicaid enrollments. Nevertheless, despite the withdrawals, commercial plans continue to play an important role in serving the Medicaid population in some markets.

The fall off in commercial plan participation has been accompanied by a rapid growth in Medicaid-only or Medicaid-dominated plans (defined as those plans that have a greater than 75 percent Medicaid enrollment). These plans vary widely in ownership type, and are a mix of for-profit and not-for-profit entities. Medicaid-only plans tend to be smaller and highly reliant on one revenue stream.

A recent study by the New York Academy of Medicine and the Columbia University School of Public Health surveyed 99 safety net plans across the country (Gray and Rowe, 2000). More than half of the entries were new plans, many of them sponsored or organized by core safety net providers. The Gray and Rowe study indicates that these plans are surviving but are "on the edge." A majority of the plans in the survey lost money in 1997 (as did many commercial plans that then exited the Medicaid market).

In assessing the impact of the current market changes, the Felt-Lisk studies suggest that little is known to date about whether and how Medicaid-only plans better serve the Medicaid population and to what degree the exit of commercial plans affects access to "mainstream" care and quality of care. However, a number of newly published studies (discussed in Chapters 4 and 5 of this report) are beginning to shed some light on this important issue.

Declining Medicaid Enrollment

After a period of steadily increasing Medicaid enrollment that began in the late 1980s, enrollment has declined steadily since 1995. Although much of this decline can be attributed to a healthy economy, shrinking Medicaid rolls have been exacerbated by the impact of welfare reform, which severed the link between cash assistance and Medicaid coverage. A 1999 analysis by the Families USA Foundation estimates that almost 700,000 people became uninsured as a direct result of welfare reform, with children making up 62 percent of those people (Families USA Foundation, 1999). A more recent U.S. General Accounting Office study measured 7 percent national decline in Medicaid enrollment between 1995 and 1997 (see Figure 3.7), ranging from only a 0.1 percent decline in Connecticut to a 17.4 percent decline in the state of Wisconsin (U.S. General Accounting Office, 1999). Counter to national trends, 10 states increased their Medicaid enrollments between 1995 and 1997. DHHS is urging states to make extra efforts to maintain Medicaid eligibility independent from eligibility for welfare assistance, but widespread difficulties in doing so remain.

The decline in Medicaid enrollment and the increased competition for some Medicaid patients in some markets are beginning to affect the revenue streams of core safety net providers (Gaskin, 1999). Eligibility and program expansions over recent years have made safety net providers increasingly reliant on Medicaid dollars. Increased Medicaid funding and cost-based reimbursement have come to provide a critical "silent subsidy" to help core safety net providers pay for overhead and infrastructure costs, freeing limited grant funds to pay for care for uninsured individuals. There are growing indications that more restricted Medicaid revenues are leaving some safety net providers in a more precarious position to fund care for the growing number of uninsured individuals seen by these providers (Solomon, 1998).

Declining Coverage for Immigrant Populations

Welfare reform has also had a serious effect on the ability of legal immigrants to gain Medicaid coverage. Provisions in the new welfare law make legal immigrants who entered the United States after August 22, 1996, ineligible for Medicaid, with the exception of emergency services, for the first 5 years after their arrival in the country. Uncertain of their rights and fearing penalties associated with applying for assistance—denial of citizenship or a "green card" to work in the United States—many immigrants continue to forego benefits to which they are legally entitled. In response, large numbers of Medicaid-ineligible documented and undocumented immigrants in states like California, Texas, New York, and Florida are placing increasing demands on already stretched safety net infrastructures. Hispanics, African Americans, and other minority groups are overrepresented among the uninsured population and make up a major segment of the safety net patient population.

In May 1999, the administration took a step to allay the fear factor, issuing a rule clarifying a long-standing "public charge" policy designed to keep immigrants from becoming dependent on government aid by denying them admission into the country or threatening deportation (Morse, 1999). Specifically, the new rule said that the State Department or Immigration and Naturalization Service may not consider Medicaid or SCHIP in deciding public charge status. The extent to which this new rule will encourage immigrants to apply for coverage is not yet known.

Declining Subsidies

Together with the eventual phaseout of FQHC cost-based reimbursement, other major direct and indirect subsidies that in the past have helped safety net providers support care for vulnerable populations are being reduced or eliminated. Since the early 1990s, safety net hospitals have increasingly relied on DSH payments to help support care for vulnerable populations. Questionable actions by states to obtain maximal DSH payments led to a tremendous rise in program expenditures, from $1.3 billion in 1990 to $17.7 billion in 1992 (Coughlin and Liska, 1998). The BBA of 1997 reduces federal DSH payments to states by $10.4 billion between fiscal years 1998 and 2002. Using data from the National Association of Public Hospitals, a new study on subsidy reductions for the core safety net underscores the critical role that DSH payments have assumed over the years in financing indigent care (Fagnani and Tolbert, 1999). In 1996 Medicare and Medicaid DSH payment combined paid for nearly 40 percent of the uncompensated care provided by core public hospitals. The report suggests that in the future DSH payment programs be better targeted to those safety net hospitals shouldering the greatest burden of uncompensated care and that the DSH payment allocation formula be reconfigured to reflect the increasing use of outpatient services.

A fundamental principle of competitive managed care is the ability of large purchasers to negotiate with MCOs for a best or discounted price for their own covered lives. These very discounts, however, which have helped slow the rate of inflation in health care costs, have also helped erode the financial margins that providers received from private payers to cover care for uninsured patients. Recent studies and surveys provide evidence that managed care cost pressures are limiting the ability of community physicians to deliver charity care (Bindman et al., 1998; Cunningham et al., 1999). Similarly, on the inpatient side, the growing penetration of Medicaid managed care and the declining ability to shift costs appear to be reducing hospitals' capacities to deliver uncompensated care (Atkinson et al., 1997; Weissman et al., 1999). Additional recent data suggest that although Medicaid revenues are being more broadly dispersed among hospitals in the 100 largest metropolitan statistical areas, uncompensated care is becoming increasingly concentrated among a smaller number of institutions (Gaskin, 1999). There is rising concern that the market is reducing the ability of the health care system to provide uncompensated care without creating a mechanism for addressing the gap in health care financing created by the decline in the level of insurance coverage (Smith, 1997).

How Core Safety Net Providers Are Responding

Although many core safety net providers were originally fearful, reluctant, and not well equipped to participate in Medicaid managed care, their rate of participation in state risk-based managed care programs has increased substantially in recent years. According to the Bureau of Primary Health Care, 437 FQHCs (nearly two-thirds) reported that they participated in Medicaid managed care arrangements in 1998, which is more than a twofold increase from the number (202) in 1995 (Bureau of Primary Health Care, HRSA, unpublished data, 1999). In many localities CHCs are viewed as attractive partners for MCOs given their locations, convenient hours, primary care orientation, and cultural and linguistic capacities (Baxter and Feldman, 1999; Lipson, 1997; West, 1999).

Growth in managed care participation now extends beyond CHCs and public hospitals to include local health departments, maternal and child health clinics, and mental health clinics (Solloway and Darnell, 1998). Many local health departments and other special service providers are facing greater hurdles in their adaptation to managed care given the more limited range of their direct service delivery component. Rural health providers, although broadly involved in managed care, face particular problems related to their special geographic and demographic characteristics (Ricketts et al., 1998).

The core safety net providers' adaptations to the new health care marketplace have brought opportunities as well as challenges. Competitive managed care has provided strong incentives for core safety net providers as well as other providers to become more efficient, more customer oriented, and more performance based. Safety net providers, however, tend to be more costly given their vulnerable and harder-to-serve patient populations, a disincentive for plans to contract with them or to pay them their costs. As mandated rather than voluntary managed care becomes predominant, many core safety net providers may be required to accept lower payments than they had received under the fee-for-service system. In addition, safety net providers generally lack the financial reserves and management and information infrastructures needed to respond quickly and competitively to the many new requirements of managed care.

Even core safety net providers that in the past resisted managed care have come to see the need to adapt to a more competitive environment. In assessing various managed care participation strategies, most safety net providers view the maintenance of their Medicaid patient base, the potential to gain greater contracting leverage in their local markets, and the ability to continue to serve the uninsured population as major priorities. Specific strategies include developing partnerships and networks; building integrated delivery systems; improving quality, customer service, and efficiency; and improving operating and information management capabilities. As a longer-term goal, core safety net providers hope to reduce dependence on Medicaid enrollment and gain Medicare and commercial contracts.

A major survey of adaptive strategies refers to the "arranged marriage" of MCOs and safety net providers. Both have valuable credentials to bring to managed care, but the challenge lies in melding often very different cultures, management styles, and service orientations (Lipson, 1997). To date, most adaptive and survival strategies are still in the early stages, and it is too early to conclude what strategies will be the most successful.

State and local policies governing care for vulnerable populations continue to be a critical dimension of how local safety nets are faring. In the past states have used "Medicaid maximization" to help protect safety net providers and to subsidize some of their services.[10] Today, a number of states are continuing to use these and other special measures aimed at either encouraging commercial health plans to include core safety net providers in their networks, facilitating the creation of managed care plans centered on core safety net providers, or providing special subsidies to major core safety net providers (Coughlin et al., 1999). There is worry, however, that these accommodations will erode potential savings to the states from Medicaid managed care. New budget priorities, unexpected

---

[10]The process of shifting state-funded programs into Medicaid and receiving a federal matching payment is commonly referred to as "Medicaid maximization" (Coughlin et al., 1999).

Medicaid cost increases, or an economic downturn could add uncertainty to the sustainability of these special provisions.

In this rapidly evolving environment, the safety net appears to be on increasingly shaky underpinnings. How current price pressures and other changes in the health care marketplace will continue to evolve and affect these providers' ability to maintain their mission to serve America's most vulnerable citizens is becoming a mounting policy concern and forms the basis of this study.

REFERENCES

Alpha Center. 1998. *Medicaid Managed Care and Safety Net Providers: A Technical Assistance Guide for Managed Care Organizations*. Princeton, NJ: Center for Health Care Strategies, Inc.

Alpha Center. 2000. *State of the States Report*. Washington, DC: Alpha Center.

Atkinson, G., Helms, W., and Needleman, J. 1997. State Trends in Hospital Uncompensated Care. *Health Affairs*, 16(4), 233–241.

Baxter, R., and Feldman, R. 1999. *Staying in the Game: Health System Change Challenges Care for the Poor*. Fairfax, VA: Center for Studying Health System Change.

Baxter, R., and Mechanic, R. E. 1997. The Status of Local Health Care Safety Nets. *Health Affairs*, 16(4), 7–23.

Bindman, A., Grumbach, K., Vranizan, K., Jaffe, D., and Osmond, D. 1998. Selection and Exclusion of Primary Care Physicians by Managed Care Organizations. *JAMA, 279*(9), 675–679.

Bovbjerg, R., and Marsteller, J. 1998. *Health Care Marketplace Competition in Six States: Implications for the Poor*. Paper No. 17. Washington, DC: The Urban Institute.

Budetti, P. 1998. Health Insurance for Children—A Model for Incremental Health Reform? *New England Journal of Medicine*, 338(8), 541–542.

Carrasquillo, O., Himmelstein, D., Woolhandler, S., and Bor, D. 1998. Can Medicaid Managed Care Provide Continuity of Care to New Medicaid Enrollees? An Analysis of Tenure on Medicaid. *American Journal of Public Health*, 88(3), 464–466.

Coughlin, T., and Liska, D. 1998. Changing State and Federal Payment Policies for Medicaid Disproportionate-Share Hospitals. *Health Affairs*, 17(3), 118–136.

Coughlin, T., Zuckerman, S., Wallin, S., and Holahan, J. 1999. A Conflict of Strategies: Medicaid Managed Care and Medicaid Maximization. *Health Services Research, 34*(1), 281–293.

Cunningham, P., and Pickreign, J. 1997. *Uninsurance Rates Vary Widely Across Communities and Regions*. Data Bulletin No. 5. Washington, DC: Center for Studying Health System Change.

Cunningham, P., and Tu, H. 1997. A Changing Picture of Uncompensated Care. *Health Affairs*, 16(4), 167–175.

Cunningham, P., Grossman, J., St. Peter, R., and Lesser, C. 1999. Managed Care and Physicians' Provision of Charity Care. *JAMA, 281*(12), 1087–1092.

Darnell, J., Rosenbaum, S., Scarpulla-Nolan, L., Zuvekas, A., and Budetti, P. 1995. *Access to Care Among Low-Income, Inner-City, Minority Populations: The Impact of Managed Care on the Urban Minority Poor and Essential Community Providers*. Washington, DC: Center for Health Policy Research, The George Washington University.

Employee Benefit Research Institute. 1999. National Health Expenditures Top $1 Trillion Dollars for Second Year in 1997. *EBRI Notes, 20*(3), 3–6.

Fagnani, L., and Tolbert, J. 1999. *The Dependence of Safety Net Hospitals and Health Systems on the Medicare and Medicaid Disproportionate Share Hospital Payment Programs.* New York, NY: The Commonwealth Fund.

Families USA Foundation. 1999. *Losing Health Insurance.* Washington, DC: Families USA Foundation.

Felt-Lisk, S., and Yang, S. 1997. Changes in Health Plans Serving Medicaid, 1993–1996. *Health Affairs, 16*(5), 125–133.

Felt-Lisk, S. 1999. *The Changing Medicaid Managed Care Market: Trends in Commercial Plans' Participation.* Washington, DC: The Henry J. Kaiser Family Foundation.

Fronstin, P. 2000. *Sources of Health Insurance and Characteristics of the Uninsured: Analysis of the March 1999 Current Population Survey.* EBRI Issue Brief No. 217. Washington, DC: Employee Benefit Research Institute.

Gaskin, D. 1999. *Safety Net Hospitals: Essential Providers of Public Health and Specialty Services.* Washington, DC: Institute for Health Care Research and Policy, Georgetown University.

Gray, B., and Rowe, C. 2000. Safety Net Health Plans: A Status Report. *Health Affairs, 19*(1), 185–193.

Gruber, J., and Levitt, L. 2000. Tax Subsidies for Health Insurance: Costs and Benefits. *Health Affairs, 19*(1), 72–85.

Henderson, T., and Markus, A. 1996. Medicaid Managed Care: How Do Community Centers Fit? *Health Care Financing Review, 17*(4), 135–142.

Holahan, J., and Liska, D. 1996. *Where Is Medicaid Spending Headed?* Washington, DC: The Urban Institute.

Holahan, J., Zuckerman, S., Evans, A., and Rangarajan, S. 1998. Medicaid Managed Care in Thirteen States. *Health Affairs, 17*(3), 43–63.

Horvath, J., Kaye, N., Pernice, C., and Mitchell, E. 1997. *Medicaid Managed Care: Program Characteristics and State Survey Results,* Vol. 1. Washington, DC: Congressional Research Service/The Library of Congress.

Hurley, R., and McCue, M. 1998. *Medicaid and Commercial HMOs: An At-Risk Relationship.* Princeton, NJ: Center for Health Care Strategies, Inc.

Hurley, R., and Wallin, S. 1998. *Adopting and Adapting Managed Care for Medicaid Beneficiaries: An Imperfect Translation.* Occasional Paper No. 7. Washington: DC: The Urban Institute.

Iglehart, J. K. 1995. Health Policy Report: Medicaid and Managed Care. *New England Journal of Medicine, 332*(25), 1727–1731.

The Kaiser Commission on Medicaid and the Uninsured. 1998a. *The Medicaid Program at a Glance.* Washington, DC: The Henry J. Kaiser Family Foundation.

The Kaiser Commission on Medicaid and the Uninsured. 1998b. *Medicaid Facts: Medicaid and Managed Care.* Washington, DC: The Henry J. Kaiser Family Foundation.

The Kaiser Commission on Medicaid and the Uninsured. 1999. *Medicaid Facts: Medicaid and Managed Care.* Washington, DC: The Henry J. Kaiser Family Foundation.

Kalkines, Arky, Zall and Bernstein, LLP. 1998. *Safety Net Plans: The Role of Provider-Sponsored Health Plans in Maintaining the Safety Net in a Managed Care Era.* New York, NY: United Hospital Fund.

Kalkines, Arky, Zall and Bernstein, LLP. 1999. *The Health Care Safety Net: Preserving Access to Care for Low-Income New Yorkers.* New York, NY: Kalkines, Arky, Zall, and Berstein, LLP.

Kaye, N., Pernice, C., and Pelletier, H. (eds.). 1999. *Medicaid Managed Care: A Guide for States,* 4th ed. Portland, ME: National Academy for State Health Policy.

Kuttner, R. 1999. The American Health Care System—Employer-Sponsored Health Coverage. *New England Journal of Medicine, 340*(3), 248–252.

Lee, J. 1997. *Managed Health Care: A Primer.* Washington, DC: Congressional Research Service/The Library of Congress.

Lefkowitz, B. and Todd, J. 1999. An Overview: Health Centers at the Crossroads. *Journal of Ambulatory Care Management, 22*(4), 1–12.

Lipson, D. 1997. Medicaid Managed Care and Community Providers: New Partnerships. *Health Affairs, 16*(4), 91–107.

Mann, J., Melnick, G., Bamezai, A., and Zwanziger, J. 1995. Uncompensated Care: Hospitals' Responses to Fiscal Pressures. *Health Affairs, 14*(1), 263–270.

Mann, J., Melnick, G., Bamezai, A., and Zwanziger, J. 1997. A Profile of Uncompensated Hospital Care, 1983–1995. *Health Affairs, 16*(4), 223–232.

McCall, N. 1996. *The Arizona Health Care Cost Containment System: Thirteen Years of Managed Care in Medicaid.* Menlo Park, CA: The Henry J. Kaiser Family Foundation.

Morse, A. 1999. CHIP and the Immigrant Community: Getting Out the Word on 'Public Charge.' *State Health Notes, 20*(308), 1, 6.

National Association of Community Health Centers. 1999. *Compromise Delays Phase-Out of Health Center Payment System—Orders Congressional Report on Impact and Alternative Payment Mechanisms.* [WWW document]. URL http://www.nachc.com/FSA/FederalAgenda/PPS/Compromise%20Announcement.htm (accessed February 1, 2000).

National Association of Public Hospitals and Health Systems. 1997. *The Balanced Budget Act of 1997: Opportunities for Safety Net Health Care Providers.* Washington, DC: National Association of Public Hospitals and Health Systems.

Norton, S., and Lipson, D. 1998. *Public Policy, Market Forces, and the Viability of Safety Net Providers.* Occasional Paper No. 13. Washington, DC: The Urban Institute.

Perry, M., Kannel, S., Valdez, R., and Chang, C. 2000. *Medicaid and Children: Overcoming Barriers to Enrollment. Findings from a National Survey.* Washington, DC: The Henry J. Kaiser Family Foundation.

Ricketts, T., Slifkin, R., and Silberman, P. 1998. Commissioned Paper. *The Changing Market, Managed Care and the Future Viability of Safety Net Providers—Special Issues for Rural Providers.* Chapel Hill, NC: Cecil G. Sheps Center for Health Services Research, University of North Carolina.

Robinson, G., Bergman, G., Crow, S., and Scallet, L. 1998. *Behavioral Health Community Providers Response to Managed Care.* Fairfax, VA: The Lewin Group.

Rosenbaum, S., and Darnell, J. 1997. *Statewide Medicaid Managed Care Demonstrations under Section 1115 of the Social Security Act: A Review of the Waiver Applications, Letters of Approval and Special Terms and Conditions.* Washington, DC: The Henry J. Kaiser Family Foundation.

Rosenbaum, S., Shin, P., Zakheim, M., Shaw, K., and Teitelbaum, J. 1998. *Negotiating the New Health System: A Nationwide Study of Medicaid Managed Care Contracts. Special Report: Mental Illness and Addiction Disorder Treatment and Prevention,* 2nd ed. Washington, DC: Center for Health Services Research and Policy, The George Washington University.

Rosenbaum, S., Shin, P., Markus, A., and Darnell, J. 2000. *A Profile of America's Health Centers.* Washington, DC: The Henry J. Kaiser Family Foundation.

Rovner, J. 1996. The Safety Net: What's Happening to Health Care of Last Resort? *Advances, Supplement*(1), 1–4. Princeton, NJ: The Robert Wood Johnson Foundation.

Schneider, A. 1997. *Overview of Medicaid Managed Care Provisions in the Balanced Budget Act of 1997.* Washington, DC: The Henry J. Kaiser Family Foundation.

Schneider, A., and Spivey, M. 1999. Commissioned Paper. *Issues in Designing a Fund for Safety Net Providers.* Washington, DC: Health Policy Group.

Shields, A. 1999. Commissioned Paper. *Understanding the Role and Future Viability of Safety Net Providers: Data Resources and Information Gaps.* Washington, DC: Institute for Health Care Research and Policy, The Georgetown University Medical Center.

Smith, B. 1997. Trends in Health Care Coverage and Financing and Their Implications for Policy. *New England Journal of Medicine, 337*(14), 1000–1003.

Solloway, M., and Darnell, J. 1998. *The Impact of Medicaid Managed Care on Essential Community Providers.* Portland, ME: National Academy for State Health Policy.

Solomon, L. 1998. Rules of the Game: How Public Policy Affects Local Health Care Markets. *Health Affairs, 17*(4), 140–148.

Thorpe, K. 1997. *The Rising Number of Uninsured Workers: An Approaching Crisis in Health Care Financing.* New Orleans, LA: Tulane University.

U.S. General Accounting Office. 1999. *Medicaid Enrollment: Amid Declines, State Efforts to Ensure Coverage After Welfare Reform Vary* (GAO/HEHS-99-163). Washington, DC: U.S. General Accounting Office.

Weissman, J., Saglam, D., Campbell, E., Causino, N., and Blumenthal, D. 1999. Market Forces and Unsponsored Research in Academic Health Centers. *JAMA, 281*(12) 1093–1098.

West, D. 1999. Medicaid Managed Care: Linking Success to Safety-Net Provider Recruitment and Retention. *Journal of Ambulatory Care Management, 22*(4), 28–32.

Zuckerman, S., Coughlin, T., Nichols, L., Liska, D., Ormond, B., Berkowitz, A., Dunleavy, M., Korb, J., and McCall, N. 1998. *Health Policy for Low-Income People in California.* Washington, DC: The Urban Institute.

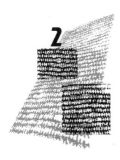

The Core Safety Net and the Safety Net System

The concept of a health care safety net conjures up the image of a tightly woven fabric of federal, state, and local programs stretched across the nation ready to catch those who slip through the health insurance system. As has already been cited in the opening chapter of this study, America's safety net is neither secure nor uniform. Rather, it varies greatly from state to state and from community to community, depending on the number of uninsured people, the local health care market, the breadth and depth of Medicaid and other programs directed at the poor and uninsured populations, as well as the general political and economic environment (Baxter and Mechanic, 1997). These variations notwithstanding, most communities can identify a set of hospitals and clinics that by mandate or mission care for a proportionately greater share of poor and uninsured people. Even within the new environment of choice and competition, these core safety net providers continue to be relied upon to play a critical role in providing access to health care for those who fall outside the market, primarily members of the nation's poorest and most disadvantaged groups.

A precise measure of the total share of care to the poor and uninsured populations delivered by safety net providers is difficult to come by, given the safety net's variability across communities, the lack of adequate and comparable data, as well as the lack of a consistent definition of the "health care safety net." Estimates show, however, that although core safety net providers such as community health centers (CHCs) and public hospitals provide a relatively small share of care to the poor and uninsured, that share is disproportionate to that provided by other health care providers. For example, 41 percent of federally qualified health center (FQHC) patients are uninsured, 33 percent are on Medicaid, 86 percent are low income, and 64 percent are people of color (Bureau of Primary Health Care, 1998). For outpatient clinics that are members of the National Association of Public Hospitals and Health Systems (NAPH),[1] 42 percent of care is to self-paying patients or patients requesting charity care and 30 percent is to Medicaid patients (National Association of Public Hospitals and Health Systems, 1999). From 1990 to 1998, FQHCs saw a 60 percent increase in the number of uninsured patients that they treated (Bureau of Primary Health Care, 1990, 1998).[2]

As part of their unique role and mission, core safety net providers offer a combination of comprehensive medical and enabling or "wrap-around" services (e.g., language interpretation, transportation, outreach, and nutrition and social support services) specifically targeted to the needs of the vulnerable populations. These services rarely generate sufficient revenues to cover their costs and are thus less likely to be provided by others in the community at large. Together with their commitment to the care for the poor and uninsured, core safety net hospitals and health systems offer critical highly specialized services such as trauma care, burn care, and neonatal care to anyone in their communities. For example, in 1997, NAPH members represented 17 percent of hospital beds in the markets but provided more than 25 percent of neonatal intensive care beds, 66 percent of burn care beds, 33 percent of pediatric intensive care beds, 45 percent of Level 1 trauma centers, and 24 percent of emergency department visits (National Association of Public Hospitals and Health Systems, 1999).

In addition, major public teaching hospitals train large numbers of physicians and other health professionals. In 1997, for example, NAPH member hospitals trained almost 16,000 residents (National Association of Public Hospitals and Health Systems, 1999).

Another major characteristic of core safety net providers is their negligible ability to shift costs, given their payer and patient mix. Cost shifting has, until recently, been a primary vehicle used by non-core safety net providers as a means of subsidizing care for the uninsured population (Cunningham et al., 1999; Davis et al., 1999). However, core safety net providers tend to have a small privately insured patient population, and

---

[1]NAPH represents over 100 safety net hospitals and health systems in metropolitan areas around the country. Most members are major teaching hospitals or academic health science centers.

[2]The 60 percent increase from 1990 to 1998 also reflects the expansion of the CHC program to include homeless and public housing programs, adding 400,000 to 500,000 users, most of whom are uninsured (Bonnie Lefkowitz, personal communication, February 2000).

unlike their non-core safety net counterparts, these providers must rely primarily on federal, state, and local grant funds and other forms of direct-subsidy payments to provide care for the poor (e.g., charitable contributions and donations) (Davis et al., 1999; Rosenbaum, 1999).

This inability to shift costs for uncompensated care onto private insurance revenues has become an even more significant problem as revenues from Medicaid, the primary source of third-party financing for the core safety net providers, are restricted. Medicaid is a central rather than marginal third-party payer for the core safety net (Rosenbaum, 1999). As a result, if future Medicaid revenues decline (whether because of a drop in the rate of coverage among the patient population or a drop in payment levels for the patient population), core safety net providers must effectively absorb this loss through the use of revenues and services intended to provide care for those without the ability to pay. Moreover, unlike private practitioners, core safety net providers cannot pass on their revenue shortfalls in the form of patient cost sharing. Not only do the patients of core safety net providers have little or no ability to pay, but the legal or mission-based obligations of the safety net providers prevent this reallocation of financial responsibilities.

Two Medicaid compensation systems—the disproportionate share hospital (DSH) payment program in the case of hospitals, and the FQHC program in the case of federally funded health centers and certain other entities—have in the past yielded Medicaid compensation levels for the core safety net that help avoid shifting costs by use of grants and subsidies intended to provide care for the uninsured population. For example, in the case of health centers, the FQHC payment structure has contributed to closer parity between health centers' Medicaid patients and their Medicaid revenues (Figure 2.1). To the extent that these payment arrangements are eliminated or reduced, core safety net providers necessarily will confront the implications of their eroding capacity to treat uninsured individuals (Felt-Lisk et al., 1997).

Against this background, this chapter provides a description of the core safety net providers and other providers in the safety net system including their patient and payer profiles, their unique structural characteristics, missions, and core competencies, and how the structures and organizations of safety net systems vary across the country.

THE HEALTH CARE SAFETY NET

Characteristics of Populations Served by the Core Safety Net

Poor people who are uninsured, are of minority and immigrant status, live in geographically or economically disadvantaged communities, or

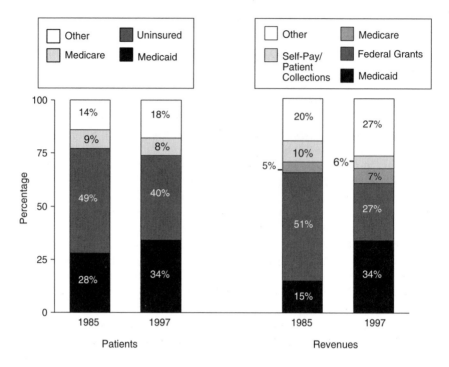

FIGURE 2.1 Changes in health center Medicaid and uninsured patients by revenue source, 1985–1997. SOURCE: The Kaiser Commission on Medicaid and the Uninsured (2000). Data from Center for Health Services Research and Policy analysis of 1997 Uniform Data System and estimates by the National Association of Community Health Centers using 1985 Bureau of Common Reporting Requirements data. Reprinted with permission of The Kaiser Commission on Medicaid and the Uninsured.

have a broad range of social, demographic, and poverty-related health problems must rely disproportionately on the core safety net for their health care (Box 2.1). For some, the primary barrier is a lack of insurance coverage. In recent years the number of uninsured individuals has grown because the cost of employment-based health insurance has become unaffordable for many low-income people and because fewer people are enrolled in Medicaid (Kronick and Gilmer, 1999). Many low-income individuals (especially Medicaid beneficiaries and low-income workers with unstable employment) move on and off of insurance. Almost two-thirds of new Medicaid enrollees lose their coverage with a year and many go on to prolonged spells without insurance (Carrasquillo et al., 1998).

BOX 2.1
The Core Safety Net Serves a Wide Range of
Vulnerable Populations

• Uninsured and underinsured

- Working poor whose employers do not offer insurance
- Non-Medicaid-covered unemployed poor
- Children who are not included in parents' coverage
- Adults who cannot afford employer-sponsored coverage

• Medicaid beneficiaries
• Chronically ill individuals
• People with disabilities
• Mentally ill individuals
• People with communicable diseases (e.g., HIV infection/AIDS or tuberculosis)
• Legal and undocumented immigrants
• Minorities
• Native Americans
• Veterans
• Homeless people
• Substance abusers
• Prisoners

SOURCE: Adapted from Gage (1998). Reprinted with permission of *The Future of the U.S. Healthcare System: Who Will Care for the Poor and Uninsured?* by S. Altman, U. Reinhardt, and A. Shields (eds.). (Chicago: Health Administration Press, 1998).

For those enrolled in Medicaid, traditionally low levels of payments to providers of health care resulted in limited and skewed provider participation, forcing many low-income patients to seek episodic care from emergency departments and hospital clinics. Medicaid coverage is often severely limited for some services such as pharmaceuticals, mental health treatment, and substance abuse treatment.

Still other populations have special needs or circumstances that can create impediments to care, such as homelessness or complex health problems, like mental illness or human immunodeficiency virus (HIV) infection/AIDS (see Chapter 6 for an expanded discussion of populations with special needs). Insurance coverage alone is often inadequate to ensure access for these populations who may require outreach and access to specialists or other support programs to meet their special needs.

Core safety net providers offer these populations a combination of essential health and social services that go beyond those provided in the commercial insurance model. Many core safety net providers have tailored their services to meet the needs of such medically underserved populations as minority communities and non-English-speaking individuals, groups that are more likely to lack insurance coverage.

Using data from the 1997 Current Population Survey and controlling for poverty and employment status, a study by The Commonwealth Fund indicated that adult minorities ages 18–64 are more likely than their white counterparts to be uninsured, suggesting that reliance on the private health insurance market may not result in substantial improvements in coverage rates for minorities (Hall et al., 1999). This means that there will continue to be a disproportionate number of minority individuals who depend on the safety net for care. A study that compared urban safety net hospitals and non-safety net hospitals in the same market areas showed dramatic concentrations of African-American and Hispanic patients at safety net hospitals relative to the concentrations at non-safety net hospitals in the market area (Gaskin, 1996) (Figure 2.2). Among public hospitals in New York City, minority patients accounted for 90 percent of outpatient visits and 88 percent of admissions in 1995 (Siegel, 1996). Similarly, nearly two-thirds of all FQHC patients in 1998 were minorities, more than 85 percent had incomes less than 200 percent of the federal poverty level and 41 percent were uninsured (Figure 2.3). More than 18 percent of the

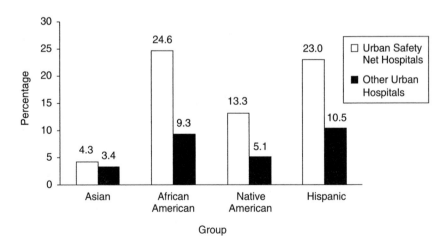

FIGURE 2.2 Ethnic and racial composition of urban safety net hospital market areas, 1994. SOURCE: Gaskin and Hadley (1999). Reprinted with permission of the Institute of Health Care Research and Policy.

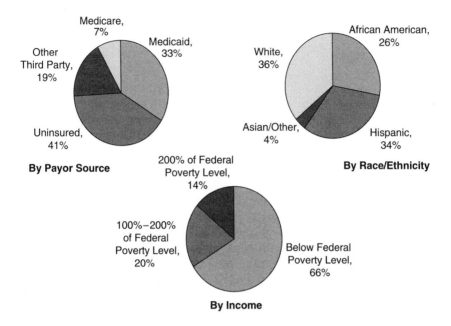

FIGURE 2.3 Payor source, income, and racial characteristics of FQHC patients, 1997. Data are based on 8.3 million users in 1997. SOURCE: 1997 Bureau of Primary Health Care Uniform Data System.

8.3 million FQHC users in 1997 required translation services; 556 of the 671 FQHCs provided translation services either directly or through a vendor (Lefkowitz, 1999). Local health departments also serve large numbers of uninsured patients, many of whom are seeking specialized services such as treatment for HIV infection/AIDS, sexually transmitted diseases (STDs), or substance abuse. Among 504 local health departments queried in a national survey conducted in March 1999, health officers estimated that one-half of urban health department clients and one-third of clients at health departments serving smaller jurisdictions were uninsured in 1998 (Shields et al., 1999). Nearly half of urban health departments and about a third of smaller health departments reported an increase in the number of uninsured clients served between January 1998 and January 1999, with the greatest increases seen among women and children.

In addition, more than 71 million Americans live in medically underserved areas (MUAs) of the country, primarily inner-city and rural areas with minimal or no economic base and very limited access to providers. According to Darnell and colleagues (1995), more than half of these people are located in urban areas and a disproportionate number are poor African-American and Hispanic individuals. In contrast, people in rural communities tend to be white but are also disproportionately poor and are underserved due to the double jeopardy created by poverty and sparse population (Kindig, 1994; Rosenbaum et al., 1998). Although these groups are highly dependent on core safety net providers, the public hospitals that serve rural communities frequently are located in distant metropolitan areas. CHCs are not evenly distributed in rural communities. Thus, vulnerable people in rural settings rely more heavily on the commitment of local providers, such as private physician practices, to maintain an open-door policy regardless of the patient's ability to pay (Ricketts et al., 1998).

Core Safety Net Providers

Core safety net providers are often referred to as "essential community providers" or "providers of last resort." As part of President Bill Clinton's health care reform initiative, the U.S. Congress in 1993 defined essential community providers as providers of health services located in federally designated MUAs or in designated health professional shortage areas or providers that are serving medically underserved populations. Such designated providers were legally obligated to provide services to the poor or were, by law, located in areas with high levels of need for health care services. Other providers who were located in underserved areas for reasons unrelated to a legal obligation (e.g., a mission to serve the poor) were not entitled to automatic designation as essential community providers. Thus, the definition made a major distinction between voluntary uncompensated care and care provided as part of a legal obligation. The Institute of Medicine's (IOM) committee's definitions of the core safety net and the safety net system have incorporated those mission-driven providers that do not meet the definition of essential community provider but that nonetheless care for a substantial share of the poor and uninsured population.

The individuals who use core safety net providers have complex needs that require both medical and enabling services, the funding for which comes from numerous sources. Over the years, Medicaid has become an increasingly important revenue source for these providers, accounting for about a third of revenues. In fact, in 1997 payments from Medicaid accounted for 33 percent of revenues for NAPH member public hospitals and 35 percent of revenues for FQHCs, whereas commercial insurers were only 10 and 9 percent, respectively (Health Resources and Services Administration, 1999; National Association of Public Hospitals and Health Systems, 1999). Thus, core safety net providers also must piece together a number of small grants from a range of federal, state, and local public and private sources to help support their missions. To highlight the patchwork quilt of safety net financing, Boxes 2.2 and 2.3 illustrate the complex funding streams for a major urban safety net provider (Denver Health, Denver, Colorado) and a rural safety-net system (Rural Health Group, Inc., Jackson, North Carolina).

Public Hospitals

There are an estimated 1,300 public hospitals in the United States (Legnini et al., 1999). Public hospitals' tradition of providing free or uncompensated care goes back more than 200 years to the early public and nonprofit charity hospitals that cared for the poorest individuals at a time when most wealthier individuals were cared for in their homes. Many functioned as charity hospitals in the nation's urban areas. These charity hospitals were outgrowths of what were once the old almshouses for the poor and provided the vulnerable citizens of cities and nearby communities with outpatient clinics, emergency services, hospitalization, and, often, dental care (Gage, 1998). Until the creation of Medicare and Medicaid in 1965, these public hospitals represented virtually the only treatment alternative available to most low-income patients.

Today, large public hospitals tend to be located in urban centers and primarily serve Medicaid beneficiaries and uninsured patients. Initially, public hospitals were owned and operated by state or local governments or public authorities. In recent years many public hospitals have closed or changed their governance to gain greater autonomy and flexibility. Some have been acquired by for-profit and not-for-profit hospital systems that may alter the roles public hospitals have been playing (see Chapter 3).

In an examination of the sources of revenue for public versus private hospitals (Table 2.1), Rosenbaum (1999) notes several key differences:

- The proportion of self-paying patients at public hospitals is far higher than that of private hospitals.
- Medicaid is a relatively marginal payer for private hospitals and a major payer for public hospitals.
- The amount of commercial coverage at public hospitals is marginal compared with that at private hospitals.
- The higher numbers of uninsured likely translates into a patient population with poorer health status compared to that of the patient population at private hospitals.

Not only is the proportion of self-paying patients much higher at public hospitals than at private hospitals but also there appears to be a big

BOX 2.2
Funding Sources for a Major Urban Safety Net Health System, Denver Health

Federal
Medicaid (Title XIX)
Medicare (Title XVIII)
Medicaid DSH payments
Medicare DSH payments
FQHC payments
Health Resources and Services Administration Bureau of Primary Health Care Section 330 Grant
Title V (Maternal and Child Health Services Block Grant)
Medicaid, Early and Periodic Screening, Diagnosis, and Treatment
Graduate Medical Education
Indirect Medical Education
Ryan White CARE Act
Medicaid Major Teaching Hospital

State
State Medicaid programs
State Children's Health Insurance Program
State medically indigent care programs
State high-risk insurance program
State public health programs
Programs to subsidize care for special populations (e.g., infants and mothers)
Programs to subsidize care for special needs of all populations (e.g., poison center grant)
Health Department's transportation funds (federal block grant)
Special Supplemental Nutrition Program for Women, Infants, and Children
Immunization Program

County
County indigent care programs
County contracts for services
Local public health programs

Other
National and state foundations
Local contributions
Self-pay
Managed care contracts
Other contracts for services
Indemnity insurance
No-fault insurance
Manufacturers' indigent drug program
Proceeds of sales and services

SOURCE: Denver Health, Denver, Colorado, 1998. Reprinted with permission.

BOX 2.3
Funding Sources for a Rural Safety Net System,
Rural Health Group, Inc.

Federal
Medicaid (Title XIX)
Medicare (Title XVII)
Child Health Insurance Programs (CHIPs) (Health Choice)
FQHC payments
Government services
    Settlement under FQHCs (cost based)
    Settlement under Rural Health Clinics (cost based)
Health Resources and Services Administration and Bureau of Primary Health Care
    Section 330 grant
    Rural Health Outreach Grant
    Rural Telemedicine (through University of North Carolina)

State
Rural obstetrical services
HIV infection/AIDS-related grant (Ryan White CARE Act)
Special Supplemental Nutrition Program for Women, Infants and Children
Special Capital Assistance Grant
Migrant Dental Program
Immunization Program
Area Health Education Center
    Clerkship Teaching Program
    Interdisciplinary Training
    Clinical Pharmacist
Upper Coastal Plains Council of Governments/Division on Aging
Area Agency on Aging
North Carolina Office of Rural Health Services
    Operational grant for five offices
    Capital grants
    Medical Assistance Program for indigents

County
Special capital assistance
Health department physician service contract

Other
Managed care companies
Indemnity insurance
Cash payments
Contracts for services
Kate B. Reynolds Charitable Trust
    Capital grants
    Indigent Medication Program grant
    Dental Expansion grant
Foundation grants
Local contributions
Manufacturers' indigent drug program

SOURCE: Rural Health Group, Inc., Jackson, North Carolina, 1998. Reprinted with permission of Thomas Irons, M.D.

TABLE 2.1 Revenue for Public Versus Private Hospitals

Type of Service	Medicare	Medicaid	Commercial	Self-Pay
Inpatient				
• Public hospital patients by payer source	20.0%	45.0%	10.0%	25.0%
• Revenues by payer source, all short-term acute care hospitals	38.0%	14.0%	38.0%	10.0%
Outpatient				
• Public hospital OPDs	13%	34%	10%	43%
• All hospital OPDs	11.6%	37.8%	32.8%	11.8%

NOTE: OPD = outpatient department. Rosenbaum (1999) encountered difficulty obtaining comparable inpatient data for public and general hospitals, thus the inpatient comparisons are between patients by payer source for public hospitals and revenues by payer source for general hospitals. In her presentation of the data, she comments that although the general hospital data would look slightly different if they were by patient rather than revenue, the differences are not large enough to significantly alter the results.

SOURCE: Rosenbaum (1999). Based on Gage (1998); unpublished data from the National Ambulatory Medical Care Expenditure Survey (1997); unpublished data from the American Hospital Association. Reprinted with permission of Sara Rosenbaum.

difference between self-paying patients at a private hospital and at a public hospital (Rosenbaum, 1999). At public facilities, self-paying patients tend to be poor and uninsured and, while they may attempt to pay part of their bill, most of the cost is absorbed by the hospital as bad debt. In contrast, at private hospitals, self-paying patients can include consumers who choose to pay for services not covered by their insurance plans.

A 1997 survey of 69 NAPH member hospitals indicated that these facilities provided more than 23 percent of the nation's uncompensated hospital care (measured as the sum of bad debt and charity care[3]) that year (National Association of Public Hospitals and Health Systems, 1999). These costs represented 26 percent of total costs at these hospitals, compared to 6 percent of total costs at the average hospital in the country. In addition, only 29 percent of these hospitals' patients had a source of insurance other than Medicaid. Therefore the ability of these urban public

---

[3]Uncompensated care is often considered an imprecise measure of the amount of care provided to low-income individuals. However, a recent study of bad-debt and free-care patients in seven Massachusetts hospitals found that most patients incurring bad debt rather than receiving charity care had incomes below the federal poverty level (Weissman et al., 1999).

hospitals to defray the costs of treating vulnerable populations is severely limited.

Public hospitals must rely on state and local government subsidies, Medicaid DSH payments, and other funds to partially offset the cost of uncompensated care. Among NAPH member hospitals in 1997, 69 percent of uncompensated care was financed by local subsidies, with an additional 22 percent financed by Medicaid DSH payments (National Association of Public Hospitals and Health Systems, 1999). These funds also underwrite the costs of providing such enabling services as translators, child care, and transportation.

In another study, the data reported by hospitals in smaller cities reveal that safety net hospitals recorded 30 percent more inpatient admissions and 39 percent more patient days than their private counterparts. Their critical role in the safety net extends to outpatient care as well, where their provision of services increased by 17.6 percent from 1988 to 1995 (National Association of Public Hospitals and Health Systems, 1997).

NAPH recently conducted an in-depth descriptive study of nine member hospital systems that included data from 25 hospitals to better understand who the uninsured are at these hospitals (Gage et al., 1998). The survey compared self-paying patients (largely indigent uninsured) with all other patients on the basis of age, sex, race, income, and service utilization.

Among the sample,[4] self-paying patients represented 40 percent of total discharges, 51 percent of total outpatient visits, and 63 percent of emergency department visits in 1996. These proportions are higher than those for the general NAPH member hospitals. Nearly 85 percent of all patients had family incomes below 150 percent of the federal poverty level. The typical uninsured patient was male (51 percent) and adult, aged 19 to 64 (78 percent). In contrast, only 59 percent of insured patients were between the ages of 19 and 64 and the majority (56 percent) were female. In the absence of national data, this targeted survey provides some useful insights into who seeks care at safety net hospitals around the nation.

Community Health Centers

Community health centers and freestanding clinics provide primary and preventative health services and tend to be located in communities whose residents have lower incomes, lack health insurance, and have less

---

[4]The surveyed hospital systems included: Boston Medical Center, Cook County Hospital (Chicago), Cooper Green Hospital (Birmingham), Denver Health Medical Center, Harris County Hospital District (Houston), Los Angeles County Department of Health Services, New York City Health and Hospitals Corporation, Parkland Health and Hospital System (Dallas), and The Regional Medical Center at Memphis.

access to health care services. Some of these centers qualify for federal funds, whereas others primarily rely on state and local government subsidies to support their missions.

Many community health centers receive federal Section 330 grant funds under the Public Health Service Act.[5] These community-based providers are also commonly referred to as FQHCs because they are qualified to receive cost-based reimbursement under Medicaid and Medicare law (see Chapter 3 for a discussion of Medicaid cost-based reimbursement). FQHC status is also extended to Native American outpatient clinics operating under Section 638 of the American Indian Self Determination Act. To be designated an FQHC, a clinic must

- be located in a medically underserved area or serve a medically underserved population;
- have nonprofit, tax exempt, or public status;
- have a Board of Directors, a majority of whom must be consumers of the center's health services;[6]
- provide culturally-competent,[7] comprehensive primary care services to all age groups;
- offer a sliding fee scale and provide services regardless of ability to pay.

In 1998, 698 FQHCs served a total of 8.7 million patients and furnished health care in all states, the District of Columbia, and the Commonwealth and Trust Territories (Bureau of Primary Health Care, 1998). The median number of health centers in a state was nine. FQHCs are not distributed evenly across the nation and range from 1 in Wyoming to 46 in California.

The number of FQHCs does not accurately reflect the actual scope of the program. In 1998, these centers reported approximately 3,000 service sites. The median number of service sites per grantee was three (Bureau of Primary Health Care, HRSA, unpublished Uniform Data System data, 1999).

Although FQHCs are divided almost equally between urban and rural

---

[5]Section 330 grant funds support traditional community health centers, migrant health centers, Health Care for the Homeless Programs, and Public Housing Primary Care Programs.

[6]This criterion is not required for homeless grantees.

[7]The Health Resources and Services Administration defines cultural competence as the ability to deliver effective medical care to people from different cultures by understanding, valuing, and incorporating the cultural differences of America's diverse population and examining one's own health-related values and beliefs (Health Resources and Services Administration, 2000).

locations, the majority of their patients reside in urban areas, mostly inner cities. All health centers provide general medical care, family planning services, outreach, social services, and immunizations to their clients; 60 percent also provide restorative dental care. In addition to the usual primary care services, migrant health centers provide special services in accident prevention and infectious and parasitic disease screening and control. Although the sizes of FQHCs vary nationwide, the average health center consists of six staff physicians, eight nurses, and three nurse practitioners or physician's assistants. Most FQHCs also employ several case managers, education specialists, and pharmacy personnel (Dievler and Giovannini, 1998).

Looking at FQHC patients by insurance status in 1998 shows that the great majority of patients were either insured by Medicaid (33 percent, or 2.84 million patients) or uninsured (41 percent, or 3.55 million patients). It is estimated that in 1998, FQHCs served approximately 9 percent of Medicaid beneficiaries, 8 percent of all the uninsured Americans, and 20 to 25 percent of the poor and near poor uninsured Americans. (Bureau of Primary Health Care, 1998).

When comparing health centers to physician practices (Table 2.2), the percentage of self-paying patients for health centers is roughly four times that of physician practices. Like public hospital patients, health center self-paying patients are more likely to be low-income uninsured individuals, whereas physician self-paying patients can range from true "charity" patients to affluent individuals who are simply not insured for a procedure. Medicaid is a large payer of health center services and a marginal payer of services provided by physicians. Therefore, any changes in Medicaid coverage levels can be expected to have a disproportionate impact on health center services (see Chapter 3).

A number of regions, cities, and counties administer and fund their

TABLE 2.2 Patients by Revenue Source: Physicians and Federally Qualified Health Centers

Type of Provider	Percentage of Patients			
	Medicare	Medicaid	Commercial	Self-Pay
Health Center	10.0	40.0	11.8	38.2
Physician practice	14.0	9.4	62.6	10.2

SOURCE: Unpublished tabulations of 1994 data by the Bureau of Primary Health Care, U.S. Department of Health and Human Services and Rosenbaum (1999), based on unpublished data from the National Ambulatory Medical Care Expenditure Survey (1994). Reprinted with permission of Sara Rosenbaum.

own freestanding primary care clinics in needy communities. For example, the San Francisco Department of Health significantly enhanced the primary care capacity for its low-income and uninsured populations by converting former public health stations into full-spectrum primary care centers. Similar efforts have occurred in Dallas (Schauffler and Wolin, 1996).

Some of these freestanding or hospital-sponsored community-based organizations have sought designation as "FQHC look-alikes." Although they do not receive federal Section 330 grant funds, they must meet FQHC eligibility criteria. Once designated they are eligible for FQHC cost-based Medicaid and Medicare payments. It is estimated that there are 124 FQHC look-alikes throughout the United States (Bureau of Primary Health Care, 1998).

This figure, however, understates the community-based safety net capacity since not every eligible provider seeks FQHC look-alike status. During the site visits the committee learned that in some states, like New York, where Medicaid already reimburses on a cost-related basis, freestanding primary care providers have no financial incentive to seek FQHC look-alike status. In fact, in such states there is a disincentive since designation as a FQHC look-alike brings with it the added costs of meeting all the Section 330 requirements.

FQHC, FQHC look-alike, and other community-based primary care clinics often rely on a patchwork of small grants to provide care for uninsured and other vulnerable patients and to support special programs (see Box 2.3). Other federal, state, local, and private programs combine to provide a significant portion of CHC grant revenues, including Title V Maternal and Child Health Block grants, Title X Family Planning grants, substance abuse treatment demonstration projects for pregnant women and children, the Healthy Start infant mortality initiative, and Title IV Ryan White CARE Act grants for primary care for people with HIV infection/AIDS. The retrieval and administration of these diverse funding sources exact heavy managerial tolls on CHCs, especially in light of their limited infrastructure resources. However, the existence of multiple funding sources can be advantageous for a center because it lessens the risk that the loss of any single source will be damaging. In addition, to survive financially, CHCs must maximize their ability to use grant, state, and local funds to support the provision of care for the uninsured population but must also maintain an adequate Medicaid revenue stream to maintain a stable fiscal base (Schauffler and Wolin, 1996).

The Rural Health Clinic (RHC) program was established in 1977 to recruit physicians, nurse practitioners, and physician's assistants in areas where Medicaid and Medicare populations were having difficulty obtaining primary care (Cheh and Thompson, 1997; U.S. General Accounting

Office, 1996). RHCs are legally obligated to serve Medicaid and Medicare beneficiaries and, in return, are entitled to cost-based reimbursement. There are nearly 2,500 federally funded RHCs that provide care to almost 4 million patients, 70 percent of whom are insured through Medicaid or Medicare (Rovner, 1996). RHCs do not have a legal obligation to provide care to uninsured individuals. In fact, there are financial disincentives to providing care to the uninsured to the degree that the provision of such care may cause the unit cost per encounter to decrease, thereby decreasing cost-based reimbursement (Ricketts et al., 1998).

More recent studies on RHCs indicated that many areas where RHCs were being certified had preexisting primary care services for the Medicaid and Medicare populations (Cheh and Thompson, 1997). The U.S. Congress, through the Balanced Budget Act of 1997 (BBA), has now restricted future RHC program growth. The new rules affect all RHCs, including those established in places where shortages of health professionals are truly severe, and are beginning to create barriers to access to primary care in some truly underserved rural areas (Ricketts et al., 1998).

Local Health Departments

The role of local health departments (LHDs) in providing direct health care services to vulnerable populations is under debate. IOM's report *The Future of Public Health* advocated that health departments focus on three core functions: assessment, assurance, and policymaking (Institute of Medicine, 1988).

Although great variations in the implementation of the core public health functions exist, all LHDs are responsible for the core public health functions listed by the U.S. Department of Health and Human Services (Baxter, 1998):

- monitor health status to identify and solve community health problems;
- diagnose and investigate health problems and hazards in the community;
- inform, educate, and empower people about health issues;
- mobilize community partnerships and action to identify and solve health problems;
- develop policies and plans that support individual and community health efforts;
- enforce laws and regulations that protect health and ensure safety;
- link people to needed personal health services and ensure the provision of health care when it is otherwise unavailable;

- ensure a competent public health and personal health care workforce;
- evaluate the effectiveness, accessibility, and quality of personal and population-based health services; and
- research new insights and innovative solutions to health problems.

According to a recent survey of 380 LHD directors, however, only 12 percent of directors believed that LHDs should be restricted to core public health functions and should provide no direct services (Keane et al., 1999).

Many of these agencies provide direct care to vulnerable populations, as well as core public health policy development and assurance functions. These services and the percentage of LHDs that provide them were summarized in a recent IOM (1998) report: immunizations, 96 percent; well-child clinic services, 79 percent; Special Supplemental Nutrition Program for Women, Infants, and Children (WIC), 78 percent; Medicaid Early Periodic Screening, Diagnosis, and Treatment (EPSDT) program, 72 percent; STD testing and counseling for STDs, 71 percent; family planning services, 68 percent; and school-based health clinics, 25 percent.

In addition, the Maternal and Child Health Bureau (MCHB), authorized under Title V of the Social Security Act, serves as a critical link in the safety net by funding health care services for mothers and children usually provided or contracted under the aegis of LHDs. Administered by the Health Resources and Services Administration, MCHB operated with a budget of $825 million in fiscal year 1997. MCHB provides services under the auspices of four major programs including (1) MCHB Block Grants, (2) Healthy Start, (3) Emergency Services for Children, and (4) HIV Coordinated Services and Access to Research (Maternal and Child Health Bureau, 1999).

Many of the more than 3,000 LHDs remain a critical source of health care for the uninsured, homeless, immigrant, and other vulnerable populations in many locales. Unlike other safety net providers, LHDs tend to specialize in providing free health care services to populations with special needs (e.g., those with HIV infection/AIDS, STDs, or drug dependence).

Changes in the delivery system and insurance market, as well as a reexamination of the role of LHDs, have led to declines in the amount of direct care provided by LHDs. The shift to managed care presents real challenges to those LHDs whose financial viability depends on revenues associated with the provision of services to Medicaid patients and other patient populations (Agency for Health Care Policy and Research, 1997). The impact of this change in policy has varied around the country. (See Chapter 3 for a more detailed description of the impacts of policy changes on LHDs.) For example, in the past the Ingham County Health Department (ICHD) of Lansing, Michigan, had the lead role in providing and ensuring the quality of federally mandated EPSDT services to both Medicaid and uninsured children. Now the program has been divided in two. One serves the Medicaid population through health maintenance organizations and the other serves the uninsured at LHDs. This has compromised ICHD's ability to conduct population-based activities that track delivery and quality of care across the entire low-income population. In Little Rock, Arkansas, loss of EPSDT activities to state-contracted health plans has resulted in a 30 percent drop in the LHD's Medicaid revenue. This has forced a reappraisal of the LHD's mission and role. On the other hand, in Cleveland, Ohio, the Cuyahoga County Board of Health is typical of LHDs that have not traditionally provided personal health services to Medicaid beneficiaries for some time. They are experiencing fewer changes as a result of Medicaid reform (Martinez and Closter, 1998). A recent study found that of 49 LHDs that provide direct care, 27 had plans to discontinue these services in favor of more traditional public health functions. Funding of city and county health departments comes predominantly from the state (40 percent) or local (37 percent) government, whereas Medicaid and categorical federal funding provide most of the remaining funds: 7 and 6 percent, respectively (Grantmakers in Health, 1998). There is no doubt that the emergence of managed care has presented LHDs with both challenges and new opportunities to use resources to carry out core public health functions. In addition, managed care has introduced the possibility that well-positioned LHDs in certain communities will develop a package of special services (e.g., school health or family planning services) that the LHD is skilled in providing and that are needed by managed care plans (Agency for Health Care Policy and Research, 1997).

Other Providers in the Safety Net System

Community and Teaching Hospitals

In most communities, the safety net includes a broader set of providers and organizations that support the delivery of health care to a variety of vulnerable populations. Although the burden for the provision of this care is highly concentrated among core safety net hospitals, many private not-for-profit hospitals either collectively or individually also provide substantial amounts of charity care and are often referred to as "the hidden health care safety net" (Altman and Guterman, 1998). Whether through emergency departments, other outpatient settings, or inpatient departments, community hospitals collectively incur approximately 60 percent of all uncompensated costs (Mann et al., 1997).

An analysis of 1994 data from the American Hospital Association's

(AHA's) Annual Survey of 5,229 community hospitals found that more than half of the hospitals in the top decile for the provision of uncompensated care were public municipal, county, hospital district, or state government entities (Fishman, 1997).[8] The top decile, however, included a substantial percentage (i.e., 46 percent) of private hospitals, among them many faith-based and private hospitals that receive little funding from state or local governments to support their charity missions. The average free-standing children's hospital, for example, devotes nearly 50 percent of its care to children who are either on Medicaid or uninsured (National Association of Children's Hospitals, 1999). These hospitals also serve as important graduate medical teaching sites.

Teaching hospitals, particularly large public teaching hospitals, are major providers of care to vulnerable populations. Teaching hospitals are often part of an academic health center (AHC) and have an affiliation with a medical school to provide clinical training. AHCs and other major teaching hospitals are often the sole providers in their communities of technologically advanced procedures for a small number of specific conditions (e.g., kidney transplants, trauma care, burn units, bone marrow transplants, and other organ transplants). Much of the uncompensated care provided by AHCs is to uninsured patients who have been transferred from other hospitals (Wyatt et al., 1997). Transferred patients have been shown to stay in the hospital twice as long as other patients, incurring double the charges.

A national study of urban academic medical centers (AMCs) reviewed their role in care for the medically underserved population, looking not only at the medically indigent but also members of minority and poor populations (Moy et al., 1996). The study confirms previous observations that these medical centers provide a large and disproportionate share of care for medically underserved members of minority and poor populations. Furthermore, the proportion of patients from these groups admitted to all urban hospitals is rising and this growth is faster among AMCs than among other hospitals. At the same time uncompensated care has also become increasingly concentrated in these teaching hospitals, particularly those under public ownership. According to AHA data, from 1989 to 1994 the share of uncompensated care provided by public teaching hospitals increased by one-third, whereas it increased by 12.4 percent among other nonteaching public hospitals (Reuter and Gaskin, 1998). In addition, 51 percent of total patient revenues for AHCs came from either Medicaid or Medicare (Blumenthal et al., 1997).

---

[8]State-owned hospitals are primarily teaching hospitals that are under common ownership with a public university.

Private Practitioners

Surveys suggest that physicians in private practice play an important collective role in the provision of care for medically indigent individuals in their communities. In a household survey conducted by the Center for Studying Health System Change, more than one-third of the uninsured who responded reported a physician's office as a usual source of care. Data collected by the American Medical Association's (AMA's) Socio-economic Monitoring System showed that uncompensated care (charity care and bad debt expenses) increased between 1990 and 1994 (Cunningham and Tu, 1997). According to the survey, in 1994 the amount of uncompensated care provided by physicians was equal to if not greater than that provided by hospitals. Although the uncompensated care provided by physicians is noteworthy, there is some evidence that for the most part private physicians tend to treat patients who are temporarily uninsured and who have incomes above 300 percent of the poverty level (Sara Rosenbaum, Washington, DC workshop testimony, May 1999; see also Table 2.2).

For the purpose of this study, three practitioner groups deserve special mention for their disproportionate contribution of care to vulnerable populations: private rural physicians, rural pharmacists, and private inner-city minority physicians.

Rural physicians are more likely than private physicians in other parts of the country to accept Medicaid or uninsured patients (Komaromy et al., 1995). Although 56 percent of physicians in nonmetropolitan areas surveyed by the AMA were full Medicaid participants,[9] the proportion dropped to 46 percent for physicians in small metropolitan areas and 41 percent for those in large metropolitan areas (Perloff et al., 1995). Among physicians in office-based practices in rural medically underserved areas, Medicaid patients account for almost 25 percent of patients (Slifkin and Crook, 1998). Although not a perfect comparison, about 12 percent of all general and family practice revenue nationwide comes from Medicaid (American Medical Association, 1998).

Private rural physicians are generally included in Medicaid managed care networks, but the extent to which these providers are losing a substantial number of insured patients to urban-based managed care is unknown (Felt-Lisk et al., 1997). Anecdotal evidence offered by rural health care providers suggests that this is occurring as large employers with primarily urban workers switch their employees, including those who

---

[9]*Full Medicaid participants* are those physicians who participate in Medicaid and accept all new Medicaid patients. In contrast, *limited participants* participate in Medicaid but accept only some new Medicaid patients or none at all (Perloff et al., 1995).

reside in rural areas, to urban managed care organizations (IOM committee conference call with rural safety net providers, October 7, 1998; see Appendix H for a full list of participants). The loss of these privately insured patients could seriously hamper the ability of rural physicians to continue to serve in their safety net role (Ricketts et al., 1998).

Rural pharmacists are the most readily accessible health professional outside metropolitan areas and are recognized as providing advice and referrals when other health care professionals are absent or scarce (American Pharmaceutical Association, 1996; Billow et al., 1991). There are signs, however, that independent rural pharmacies are disappearing as the industry becomes characterized by chain pharmacies, which are usually located in larger retail stores and shopping centers, and by mail-order pharmacy services (Gangeness, 1997; Smith and Coons, 1990). State studies indicate that although access is only marginally lower, existing rural pharmacies are showing marked declines in profit levels and financial viability (Straub and Straub, 1998). It may be only a matter of time before access to pharmacies and pharmacy-related services becomes a more serious problem in rural areas.

In their report to The Commonwealth Fund, Darnell and colleagues (1995) take special note of the role played by inner-city minority physicians in the care of poor and uninsured individuals. Studies have found that these physicians are more likely to care for patients who are racial and ethnic minorities, Medicaid beneficiaries, and uninsured (Moy and Bartman, 1995). Surveys have shown that more than half of minority medical students would prefer to practice in large cities and that 40 percent (compared with only 9 percent of nonminority students) planned to practice in socioeconomically deprived areas (Association of American Medical Colleges, 1994).

There is some anecdotal evidence that some minority physicians are finding it more difficult to enter managed care arrangements (Darnell et al., 1995; Mackenzie et al., 1998). The only known systematic evaluation of this issue (Bindman et al., 1998) was conducted in California, using a mail survey of a sample of physicians providing primary care in the state's 13 largest urban counties. The study found no statistical evidence that minority physicians were disproportionately experiencing denials or terminations in managed care contracting. The study suggests, however, that managed care plans may be more reluctant to contract with office-based physicians who provide a greater share of charity care. In the absence of comparable assessments from other parts of the country, concern remains that the special role of key providers serving vulnerable inner-city populations may be uniquely threatened by the growth of managed care.

School-Based Health Centers

The first school-based centers were established in the early 1970s to ensure quality health care for all school-age children regardless of their families' socioeconomic status. Since the 1990s, school-based health centers have proliferated. According to a recent survey, the number of school-based health centers in the United States in 1998 had increased to 1,157, almost double the number in 1994 (The Robert Wood Johnson Making the Grade Program Office, 1998). Of the 40 school-based clinics participating in the Robert Wood Johnson Foundation Making the Grade Program, 63 percent are in urban areas, with a little more than half in elementary schools or schools for kindergarten through grade 12; the rest are in middle schools and high schools. Almost 70 percent operate full time (defined as 25 hours a week). School-based centers provide physical and behavioral health care interventions and use multidisciplinary teams of nurse practitioners, physicians, and social workers. Traditionally, these centers have relied on private funds as well as federal, state, and local grants. Sponsorship is 20 percent hospital, 25 percent CHC, 20 percent LHD, 10 percent school district, 10 percent community-based organization, and 15 percent school health care organization (The Robert Wood Johnson Making the Grade Program Office, 1998). Recently, however, they have turned to third-party reimbursement, in particular, Medicaid managed care plans, as a source of revenue. Many believe that the State Children's Health Insurance Program will be another promising source of funding. Yet, there are continuing concerns about the financial sustainability of school-based centers (Friedrich, 1999). According to the Making the Grade Program survey, federal funding for school-based clinics has declined by $2.5 million since 1996.

The locations of school-based clinics—63 percent are in urban areas—and their emphases on behavioral as well as physical health make these clinics attractive sources of care for newly insured children. Clinics in 38 states are eligible for Medicaid reimbursement, and 25 states have encouraged the clinics to participate in Medicaid managed care. About half of the states have established standards of operation, and seven states license school-based clinics (The Robert Wood Johnson Foundation Making the Grade Program Office, 1998).

Federally Sponsored Health Services

Although not the subject of this study, the committee wishes to acknowledge the roles of the Veteran Health Administration (VHA) and the Indian Health Service (IHS) in the provision of care to the poor and uninsured individuals. These providers care for about 4 million veterans and Native Americans and Alaska Natives, many of whom might otherwise add to the demand on the core safety net.

The original mission of the VHA was to provide hospital care for veterans with service-connected disabilities. Over the years this mission has expanded to include both inpatient and outpatient care for veterans with service-connected disabilities and for veterans with non-service-connected disabilities (National Health Policy Forum, 1998).

Veterans Affairs (VA) hospitals and ambulatory care services are often an unrecognized but significant source of safety net services. In fact, the VA medical center system is one of the nation's largest health care systems, with 173 hospitals, 600 outpatient clinics, 133 nursing homes, 40 domiciliaries, 206 counseling centers, and 185,000 employees. Each year these facilities serve approximately 10 percent of the total veteran population, providing comprehensive services to approximately 2.5 million veterans annually. Only about 12 percent of those treated at a VA facility are treated for a service-connected disability. The majority are poor; 70 percent have annual incomes less than $21,610 (National Health Policy Forum, 1998).

IHS works in conjunction with 547 federally recognized tribes to deliver health care to Native Americans and Alaska Natives throughout the country. IHS is the primary, and often the sole, provider of health services for many Native Americans and Alaska Natives. IHS has a staff of 14,500 that operates with approximately $2.2 billion in federal appropriations and that serves 1.4 million beneficiaries in 500 direct care centers. In addition, IHS operates the Contract Health Services program with non-IHS providers, which currently accounts for 18 percent of all expenditures. Although direct and contracted patient care is a large component of IHS, it also provides environmental and educational services. Hospital and ambulatory care, preventive services, and alcohol treatment account for most of the IHS expenditures on direct services. IHS provides services through a broad range of facilities and personnel: 37 IHS hospitals, including 3 major medical centers; 64 health centers; 5 school-based health centers; 50 health stations; and an array of physicians, dentists, nurses, pharmacists, and other health care professionals (Indian Health Service, 1997).

THE SPECIAL VALUE OF CORE SAFETY NET PROVIDERS

As health care continues its transformation toward a more market-oriented, performance-based system, special treatment for designated classes of providers—even those providers with important social missions—will be highly dependent on their proven ability to add value and operate efficiently. Despite their laudable track record for caring for disproportionate numbers of this nation's poorest and sickest population groups, core safety net providers are often viewed as operating in a less efficient manner than other groups of providers and with less ability to document their unique contributions to health outcomes for their patient populations (Harrington et al., 1998; Thorpe and Brecher, 1987). In addition, the committee heard and read evidence that safety net hospitals and clinics operated by state, municipal, or other government subdivisions may be at a disadvantage in their ability to make timely business decisions, form strategic partnerships, or succeed in a more competitive environment given the hiring, procurement, and other rules with which such publicly owned entities have to comply (Bovbjerg and Marsteller, 1998; Siegel, 1996; West, 1999). Evaluations of safety net providers in some of the states that have received 1115 waivers found that many of these providers have weak existing business and administrative functions largely because the bulk of their business has been limited to the Medicaid, Medicare, and uninsured populations, none of which required strong business skills (Hoag et al., 1999). In a system of surplus capacity and downsizing, the ability to measure and demonstrate competitive financial and quality performance is becoming a critical requirement for future survival, for both private and traditionally publicly sponsored health care providers.

Although concerns about inefficiencies are occasionally cited, the committee found very limited evidence with which to assess the relative efficiency of safety net providers. The majority of articles devoted to this issue point to safety net providers' more complex patient population and the broader array of services that they have to offer. These "product" differences make assessments of comparative efficiency more difficult (Landon and Epstein, 1999; Lipson, 1997; Savela et al., 1998; Schauffler and Wolin, 1996).

The move to a more market-based system has called renewed attention on issues of efficiency and effectiveness in health care. The phaseout of cost-based reimbursement for FQHCs in the 1997 BBA was propelled in part by a perception in the U.S. Congress and among state governors that such cost-based reimbursement provides few incentives for efficient behavior. A 1998 study with data from 328 health centers assessed the impact of cost-based reimbursement for FQHCs on revenue and utilization. Although the sample was not perfectly representative of all CHCs, the study demonstrated that the shift to cost-based reimbursement increased the total number of users and Medicaid beneficiaries who receive care at CHCs but that there was no direct link to overall increases in medical encounters per user. The focus on volume is important because states are already allowed to apply caps and productivity screens to the per visit rate (Lewis-Idema et al., 1998).

However, some policy makers contend that despite the potential for internal controls, the cost-related payment system of FQHC is not consistent with an emphasis on managed care. Therefore, a number of bills were introduced in the 106th U.S. Congress to develop some type of prospective payment system for FQHCs to replace the current cost-based reimbursement system. Lack of agreement on a new method led to the BBA Refinements Act of 1999, which tempered the cost reimbursement phaseout as outlined in the 1997 BBA and called for a study to assess alternative payment strategies.

Unresolved payment issues aside, studies have demonstrated that these providers can be uniquely effective in addressing the special needs of certain vulnerable populations (Andrulis and Goodman, 1999; Rosenbaum et al., 2000). For example, New York City's Health and Hospital Corporation, the country's largest public hospital system, serves about 55 percent of the city's patients with AIDS, 48 percent of its patients with tuberculosis, and about 36 percent of its patients who need inpatient psychiatric treatment (LaRay Brown, Health and Hospital Corporation, personal communication, March 2000). A study to assess whether the presence of a public hospital in a community increased access to care among the poor found that the presence of such a hospital not only increased the volume of care provided to the medically indigent population, but also reduced the uncompensated care burden for private hospitals (Thorpe and Brecher, 1987). The study also found that public hospitals in cities with a substantial level of graduate medical education delivered proportionately more uncompensated care than nonteaching public hospitals. A 1990 study by Bindman and colleagues found that the closing of a public hospital in a semirural area of northern California had a significant effect on access to health care and was associated with a decline in the self-reported health status of patients previously served by the closed hospital (Bindman et al., 1990).

A number of comprehensive literature reviews of CHCs and the Medicaid program have documented that the effectiveness and cost-effectiveness of CHCs in improving access to ambulatory care, reducing inappropriate hospitalizations, and delivering quality care, was comparable to that of other types of providers (Davis and Schoen, 1977; Dievler and Giovannini, 1998; Hawkins and Rosenbaum, 1998). A study that looked at the impact on access to health care after the introduction of CHCs in five low-income areas across the country found that the availability of CHCs not only increased access to medical and dental care but also resulted in a major shift in care from hospital clinics to CHCs and a significant reduction in hospital inpatient use (Okada and Wan, 1980). The new CHCs also attracted people with no previous source of care. The study found, however, that although Medicaid and the presence of CHCs greatly facilitated the use of health services, disparity in the utilization of health and dental care remained between the study areas and the averages for the nation. The impact of health centers on outcomes was demonstrated by a national analysis of county data using multivariate techniques which attributed 12 percent of the decline in black infant mortality from 1970 to 1977 to the presence of CHCs (Goldman and Grossman, 1988).

A seminal study by a team of researchers at the Johns Hopkins School of Hygiene and Public Health that looked at the relationship between efficiency in the use of resources and quality of care in different primary care settings targeted mainly to Medicaid beneficiaries found that, irrespective of costs, the quality of medium-cost health centers met or exceeded the quality of other providers (Starfield et al., 1994). Another study by a Johns Hopkins-based team compared Medicaid utilization and expenditures for users of health centers and other providers and found that, after adjusting for case mix, health center users had costs and inpatient admissions similar to those for patients who used private physicians for their primary care and less than those who used hospital clinics (Stuart and Steinwachs, 1993). A more recent but related study on income, inequality, primary care, and health indicators, also conducted by researchers at Johns Hopkins, found that availability of primary care may in part help overcome the severe adverse impact of income inequalities on health (Shi et al., 1999).

Other recent analyses found that Medicaid users of CHCs experience a 22 percent lower rate of hospitalization for ambulatory care sensitive conditions than Medicaid beneficiaries who receive medical services from other primary care providers (Falik et al., 1998). A nationally representative survey of health center patients conducted by Mathematica Policy Research, Inc. in 1995 for the Bureau of Primary Health Care found that female health center patients are more likely to obtain mammographies, clinical breast exams, and Pap smear tests than a comparison group drawn from the National Health Interview Survey (Regan et al. 1999). Moreover, both this study and a survey for the Picker-Commonwealth Fund based on a representative sample of health center patients reported high levels of satisfaction, respectful treatment, increased access over other providers, convenient hours, and availability of translation/interpretation into their own language (Regan et al., 1999; Zuvekas et al., 1999).

A longitudinal study on the impact of pediatric visits to hospital emergency departments after the establishment of a neighborhood health center found that inappropriate emergency department visits declined significantly with the establishment of the center in a poor Rochester, New York, neighborhood (Hochheiser et al., 1971). No such decline was observed among residents of a control community that remained without a CHC. The study suggests, however, that the proximity of underserved populations to health services is an important but not an overriding inducement to use. Access and provision of quality care for poverty residents, the study shows, must be associated with aggressive outreach, cultural considerations, and effective communications.

A study that looked at the effects of Florida's Medicaid eligibility expansions for pregnant women found that access and birth outcomes improved for low-income women who did not have private insurance (Long and Marquis, 1998). These improvements in access and outcome were linked to the availability of county health department services. Study results showed the importance of linking expanded insurance coverage for low-income women with a delivery system that can accommodate their special needs. However, a study by researchers at the Agency for Health Care Policy and Research and the University of California challenged these findings and showed that Medicaid-eligible women who obtained multidisciplinary prenatal care at private physician's offices that were reimbursed by Medicaid for enhanced care had equal or better outcomes than women served by local health departments (Simpson et al., 1997).

A more recent study from California sheds additional light on this issue. Using telephone surveys of residents in urban California communities, Grumbach and colleagues found that physician supply alone may not guarantee effective access to care for disadvantaged populations (Grumbach et al., 1997). The study suggests that in poor communities physician supply may need to be linked with organizational structures that address the multiple sociodemographic factors that can impede access to care.

SAFETY NET PROVIDERS IN A CHANGING HEALTH CARE ENVIRONMENT

Today's environment of change and challenge will likely have important policy and program implications for the nation's traditional safety net providers. As the rolls of the uninsured continue to expand, other major players in the delivery system are finding it more difficult to sustain their past commitment to uncompensated care, placing more of the burden on public hospitals and CHCs. Despite this reliance and the acknowledged contributions of safety net providers, profound questions are being raised today about how the future financing of health care and health care for poor and uninsured individuals should be organized and funded. Devolution and the market paradigm with its dynamics of competition, consumerism, and choice have focused major interest in expanding access to affordable insurance for low-income Americans as an alternative to continued government support for a designated set of providers.

Whereas core safety net providers have always survived on a tenuous patchwork of funding, the policy and political mindsets in many quarters support the notion that these, as well as other providers, should be challenged to operate more effectively and efficiently even with more limited resources and with patients with more complicated medical conditions and socioeconomic challenges.

The committee concludes that the safety net system is a distinct delivery system, however imperfect, that addresses the needs of the nation's most vulnerable populations. In the absence of total reform of the health care system and while the new market paradigms are unfolding, it seems likely that the nation will continue to rely on safety net providers to care for its most vulnerable and disadvantaged populations. Chapter 3 provides a comprehensive analysis of the major factors that affect the health care safety net.

REFERENCES

Agency for Health Care Policy and Research. 1997. *Local Health Departments in a Managed Care Environment: Challenges and Opportunities.* Workshop Summary, May 6–8, 1997, User Liaison Program. [WWW document]. URL http://www.ahcpr.gov/research/ulplocmc.htm (accessed September 18, 1998).

Altman, S., and Guterman, S. 1998. The Hidden U.S. Healthcare Safety Net: Will It Survive? In: *The Future U.S. Healthcare System: Who Will Care For the Poor and Uninsured?* Altman, S., Reinhardt, U., and Shields, A. (eds.) Chicago, IL: Health Administration Press; pp. 167–186.

American Medical Association. 1998. *Physician Marketplace Statistics.* Chicago, IL: Center for Health Policy Research, American Medical Association.

American Pharmaceutical Association. 1996. Studies Affirm Pharmacists as the Most Accessible Part of Rural Health Care. *Pharmacy Today,* 2(4), 1–2.

Andrulis, D., and Goodman, N. 1999. *The Social and Health Landscape of Urban and Suburban America.* Chicago, IL: Health Forum.

Association of American Medical Colleges. 1994. *Minority Students in Medical Education: Facts and Figures VIII.* Washington, DC: Association of American Medical Colleges.

Baxter, R. 1998. The Roles and Responsibilities of Local Public Health Systems in Urban Health. *Journal of Urban Health: Bulletin of the New York Academy of Medicine,* 75(2), 322–329.

Baxter, R., and Mechanic, R.E. 1997. The Status of Local Health Care Safety Nets. *Health Affairs,* 16(4), 7–23.

Billow, J.A., Van Riper, G.C., Baer, L.L., and Stover, R.G. 1991. The Crisis in Rural Pharmacy Practice. *American Pharmacy,* NS31, 51–53.

Bindman, A., Keane, D., and Lurie, N. 1990. A Public Hospital Closes: Impact on Patients' Access to Care and Health Status. *JAMA,* 264(22), 2899–2904.

Bindman, A., Grumbach, K., Vranizan, K., Jaffe, D., and Osmond, D. 1998. Selection and Exclusion of Primary Care Physicians by Managed Care Organizations. *JAMA,* 279(9), 675–679.

Blumenthal, D., Campbell, E.G., and Weissman, J.S. 1997. *Understanding the Social Missions of Academic Health Centers.* New York, NY: The Commonwealth Fund.

Bovbjerg, R., and Marsteller, J. 1998. *Health Care Market Competition in Six States: Implications for the Poor*, Paper Number 17. Washington, DC: The Urban Institute.

Bureau of Primary Health Care. 1990. Unpublished tabulations based on grant applications. Bethesda, MD: Bureau of Primary Health Care/Health Resources and Services Administration, U.S. Department of Health and Human Services.

Bureau of Primary Health Care. 1998. Uniform Data System. Bethesda, MD: Bureau of Primary Health Care/Health Resources and Services Administration, U.S. Department of Health and Human Services.

Carrasquillo, O., Himmelstein, D., Woolhandler, S., and Bor, D. 1998. Can Medicaid Managed Care Provide Continuity of Care to New Medicaid Enrollees? An Analysis of Tenure on Medicaid. *American Journal of Public Health, 88*(3), 464–466.

Cheh, V., and Thompson, R. 1997. *Rural Health Clinics: Improved Access at a Cost*. Contract Report to Office of Research and Demonstrations, Health Care Financing Administration. Princeton, NJ: Mathematica Policy Research, Inc.

Cunningham, P., Grossman, J., St. Peter, R., and Lesser, C. 1999. Managed Care and Physician's Provision of Charity Care. *JAMA 281*(12), 1087–1092.

Cunningham, P., and Tu, H. 1997. A Changing Picture of Uncompensated Care. *Health Affairs 16*(4), 167–175.

Darnell, J., Rosenbaum, S., Scarpulla-Nolan, L., Zuvekas, A., and Budetti, P. 1995. *Access to Care Among Low-Income, Inner-City, Minority Populations: The Impact of Managed Care on the Urban Minority Poor and Essential Community Providers*. Washington, DC: Center for Health Policy Research, The George Washington University.

Davis, K., Collins, K., and Hall, A. 1999. *Community Health Centers in a Changing U.S. Health Care System*. New York, NY: The Commonwealth Fund.

Davis, K., and Schoen, C. 1977. *Health and the War on Poverty: A Ten-Year Appraisal*. Washington, DC: The Brookings Institution.

Dievler, A., and Giovannini, T. 1998. Community Health Centers: Promise and Performance. *Medical Care Research and Review, 55*(4), 405–431.

Falik, M., Needleman, J., Korb, J., and McCall, N. 1998. *ACSC Experience by Usual Source of Care: Comparing Medicaid Beneficiaries, CHC-Users and Comparison Groups*. Wheaton, MD: MDS Associates.

Felt-Lisk, S., Harrington, M., and Aizer, A. 1997. *Medicaid Managed Care: Does it Increase Primary Care Services in Underserved Areas?* Washington, DC: Mathematica Policy Research, Inc.

Fishman, L.E. 1997. What Types of Hospitals Form the Safety Net? *Health Affairs, 16*(4), 215–222.

Friedrich, M.J. 1999. 25 Years of School-Based Health Centers. *JAMA, 281*(9), 781–782.

Gage, L. 1998. The Future of Safety Net Hospitals. *In: The Future of the U.S. Healthcare System: Who Will Care for the Poor and Uninsured?*, Altman, S., Reinhardt, U., and Shields, A. (eds.). Chicago, IL: Health Administration Press.

Gage, L., Fughani, L., Tolbert, J. and Capito-Burch, C. 1998. *America's Uninsured and Underinsured: Who Cares?* Washington, DC: National Association of Public Hospitals.

Gangeness, D.E. 1997. Pharmaceutical Care for Rural Patients: Ominous Trends. *Journal of the American Pharmaceutical Association, NS37*, 62–65, 84.

Gaskin, D. 1996. The Impact of Managed Care and Public Safety Policy Changes on Urban Safety Net Hospitals. Working Paper. Washington, DC: Institute for Health Care Research and Policy, Georgetown University.

Gaskin, D., and Hadley J. 1999. Population Characteristics of Safety Net and Other Urban Hospitals' Markets. *Journal of Urban Health: Bulletin of the New York Academy of Medicine, 76*(3), 351–370.

Goldman, F., and Grossman, M. 1988. The Impact of Public Health Policy: The Case of Community Health Centers. *Eastern Economic Journal*, 14(1), 63–72.

Grantmakers in Health. 1998. *As the New Millennium Dawns—Will Public Health Agencies Be Up to the Challenge of Ensuring the Public's Health?* GIH Bulletin: Safety Net Focus. February 23, 1998: Grantmakers in Health.

Grumbach, K., Vranizan, K., and Bindman, A. 1997. Physician Supply and Access to Care in Urban Communities. *Health Affairs, 16(1)*. 71–86.

Hall, A.G., Collins, S.C., Glied, S. 1999. *Employer Sponsored Health Insurance: Implication for Minority Workers* [WWW document]. URL http//www.cmwf.org/programs/minority/hall_minorityinsur_ 314.asp #executive_ (accessed February 11, 2000).

Harrington, M., Frazer, H., and Aizer, A. 1998. *Medicaid Managed Care and FQHCs: Experiences of Plans, Networks, and Individual Health Centers.* Washington, DC: Mathematica Policy Research, Inc.

Hawkins, D., and Rosenbaum, S. 1998. The Challenges Facing Health Centers in a Changing Healthcare System. *In: Who Will Take Care of the Poor and Uninsured?*, Altman, S., Reinhardt, U., and Shields, A. (eds.). Chicago, IL: Health Administration Press.

Health Resources and Services Administration. 1999. Unpublished tabulations of Uniform Data System data. Rockville, MD: Health Resources Services Administration, U.S. Department of Health and Human Services.

Health Resources and Services Administration. 2000. Health Care Rx: Access for All [WWW document]. URL: http://www.hrsa.dhhs.gov/newsroom/ features.htm (accessed February 18, 2000).

Hoag, S., Norton, S., and Rajan, S. 1999. *Effects of Medicaid Managed Care Demonstrations on Safety Net Providers in Hawaii, Rhode Island, Oklahoma, and Tennessee.* Princeton, NJ: Mathematica Policy Research, Inc.

Hochheiser, L., Woodward, K., and Charney, E. 1971. Effect of the Neighborhood Health Center on the Use of Pediatric Emergency Departments in Rochester, NY. *New England Journal of Medicine, 285(3)*, 148–152.

Indian Health Service. 1997. *Profile and Mission Statement*, March 18, 1997. Washington, DC: Indian Health Service, Public Health Service, U.S. Department of Health and Human Services.

Institute of Medicine. 1988. *The Future of Public Health.* Washington, DC: National Academy Press

Institute of Medicine. 1998. *America's Children: Health Insurance and Access to Care.* Washington, DC: National Academy Press.

The Kaiser Commission on Medicaid and the Uninsured. 2000. *Health Centers' Role as Safety Net Providers for Medicaid Patients and the Uninsured.* Washington, DC: The Henry J. Kaiser Family Foundation.

Keane, C., Marx, J., and Ricci, E. 1999. Privatization and the Scope of Public Health: A National Survey of Local Health Departments. Working paper. Graduate School of Public Health, University of Pittsburgh, Pittsburgh, PA, August 19, 1999.

Kindig, DA. 1994. *Medical Underservice in Rural America in a Changing Health Care System.* Washington, DC: The Henry J. Kaiser Family Foundation.

Komaromy, M., Lurie, N., and Bindman, A.B. 1995. California Physicians' Willingness to Care for the Poor. *Western Journal of Medicine, 162*, 127–132.

Kronick, R., and Gilmer, T. 1999. Explaining the Decline in Health Insurance Coverage, 1979–1995. *Health Affairs, 18(2)*, 30–47.

Landon, B., and Epstein, A. 1999. Quality Management Practices in Medicaid Managed Care: A National Survey of Medicaid and Commercial Health Plans Participating in the Medicaid Program. *JAMA, 282(18)*, 1769–1775.

Lefkowitz, B. 1999. Unpublished tabulations of annual data reported to Bureau of Primary Health Care, Health Resource Services Administration, U.S. Department of Health and Human Services, Bethesda, MD.

Legnini, M., Anthony, S., Wicks, E., Meyer, J., Rybowski, L., and Stepnick, L. 1999. *Summary of Findings: Privatization of Public Hospitals.* Washington, DC: The Henry J. Kaiser Family Foundation.

Lewis-Idema, D., Chu, R., Hughes, R., and Lefkowitz, B. 1998. FQHC: Harnessing the Incentives of Cost Reimbursement. *Journal of Ambulatory Care Management, 21*(2), 58–75.

Lipson, D. 1997. Medicaid Managed Care and Community Providers: New Partnerships. *Health Affairs, 16*(4), 91–107.

Long, S., and Marquis, S. 1998. The Effects of Florida's Medicaid Eligibility Expansion for Pregnant Women. *American Journal of Public Health, 88*(3), 371–376.

Mackenzie, E., Taylor, L., and Lavizzo-Mourey, R. 1998. Experiences of Ethnic Minority Primary Care Physicians with Managed Care: A National Survey. *American Journal of Managed Care, 5*(10), 1251–1264.

Mann, J., Melnick, G., Bamezai, A., and Zwanziger, J. 1997. A Profile of Uncompensated Hospital Care, 1983–1995. *Health Affairs, 16*(4), 223–232.

Martinez, R.M. and Closter, E. 1998. Public Health Departments Adapt to Medicaid Managed Care. Issue Brief 16. Washington, DC: Center for Studying Health Systems Change.

Maternal and Child Health Bureau. 1999. *Maternal and Child Health Bureau—Overview.* [WWW document]. URL http://www.hhs.gov/hrsa/mchb/overview.htm (accessed January 10, 1999).

Moy, E., and Bartman, B. 1995. Physician Race and Care of Minority and Medically Indigent Patients. *JAMA, 273*(19), 1515–1520.

Moy, E., Valente, E., Jr., Levin, R.J., and Griner, P.F. 1996. Academic Medical Centers and the Care of Underserved Populations. *Academic Medicine, 71*(12), 1370–1377.

National Association of Children's Hospitals. 1999. About NACH [WWW document]. URL http://www.childrenshospitals.net/nach/about/ about_index.html (accessed December 23, 1999).

National Association of Public Hospitals and Health Systems. 1997. Preserving America's Safety Net Health Systems: An Agenda for Federal Action. Washington, DC: National Association of Public Hospitals and Health Systems.

National Association of Public Hospitals and Health Systems. 1999. *America's Safety Net Hospitals and Health Systems.* Washington, DC: National Association of Public Hospitals and Health Systems.

National Health Policy Forum. 1998. *Restructuring the VA Health Care System: Safety Net, Training, and Other Considerations,* pp. 2–14. Issue Brief No. 716. Washington, DC: The George Washington University.

Okada, L., and Wan, T. 1980. Impact of Community Health Centers and Medicaid on the Use of Health Services. *Public Health Reports, 95*(6), 520–534.

Perloff, J.D., Kletke, P., and Fossett, J.W. 1995. Which Physicians Limit Their Medicaid Participation and Why. *Health Services Research, 30*(1), 7–26.

Regan, J., Lefkowitz, B., and Gaston, M. 1999. Cancer Screening among Community Health Center Women: Eliminating the Gaps. *Journal of Ambulatory Care Management, 22*(4), 45–52.

Reuter, J., and Gaskin, D., 1998. The Role of Academic Health Centers and Teaching Hospitals in Providing Care for the Poor. *In: The Future of the U.S. Healthcare System: Who Will Care for the Poor and Uninsured?* Altman, S., Reinhardt, U., and Shields, A. (eds.). Chicago, IL: Health Administration Press, pp. 151–165.

Ricketts, T.C., Slifkin, R.T., and Silberman, P. 1998. Commissioned Paper. The Changing Market, Managed Care and the Future Viability of Safety Net Providers—Special Issues for Rural Providers. Chapel Hill, NC: The University of North Carolina, Cecil G. Sheps Center for Health Services Research.

Rosenbaum, S. 1999. Changing Public Policy and the Viability of the Safety Net. Paper presented at the Workshop on the Safety Net in a Changing Environment, Washington, DC, April 19, 1999.

Rosenbaum, S., Hawkins, Jr., D.R., Rosenbaum, E., and Blake, S. 1998. State Funding of Comprehensive Privacy Medical Care Service Programs for Medically Underserved Populations. *American Journal of Public Health, 88*(3), 357–363.

Rosenbaum, S., Shin, P., Markus, A., and Darnell, J. 2000. A Profile of America's Health Centers. Washington, DC: The Henry J. Kaiser Family Foundation.

Rovner, J. 1996. The Safety Net: What's Happening to Health Care of Last Resort? *Advances,* Supplement, (1), 1–4. Princeton, NJ: The Robert Wood Johnson Foundation.

Savela, T., Chimento, L., and Stacy, N. 1998. *The Performance of C/MHCs Under Managed Care: Case Studies of Seven C/MHCs and their Lessons Learned.* Fairfax, VA: The Lewin Group.

Schauffler, H.H., and Wolin, J. 1996. Community Health Clinics Under Managed Competition: Navigating Uncharted Waters. *Journal of Health Politics, Policy and Law, 21*(3), 460–488.

Shi, L., Starfield, B., Kennedy, B., and Kawachi, I. 1999. Income Inequality, Primary Care, and Health Indicators. *Journal of Family Practice, 48*(4), 275–284.

Shields, A., Peck, M., and Sappenfield, W. 1999. Local Health Departments and the Health Care Safety Net. Working Paper. Washington, DC: Institute for Health Care Research and Policy, Georgetown University.

Siegel, B. 1996. *Public Hospitals—A Prescription for Survival.* New York, NY: The Commonwealth Fund.

Simpson, L., Korenbrot, C., and Greene, J. 1997. Outcomes of Enhanced Prenatal Services for Medicaid-Eligible Women in Public and Private Settings. *Public Health Reports, 112,* 122-132.

Slifkin, R., and Crook, K. 1998. Unpublished analysis of rural physician survey data. Rural Health Research Program, Cecil G. Sheps Center for Health Services Research, University of North Carolina at Chapel Hill.

Smith, H.A., and Coons, S.J. 1990. Patronage Factors and Consumer Satisfaction with Sources of Prescription Purchases. *Journal of Pharmaceutical Marketing and Management, 4*(3), 61–80.

Starfield, B., Powe, N., Weiner, J., Stuart, M., Steinwachs, D., Scholle, S., and Gerstenberger, A. 1994. Costs vs. Quality in Different Types of Primary Care Settings. *JAMA, 272*(24), 1903–1908.

Straub, L.A., and Straub, S.A. 1998. Unpublished Manuscript. Consumer and Provider Evaluation of Rural Pharmacy Services. Department of Economics, Western Illinois University, Macomb.

Stuart, M.E., and Steinwachs, D.M. 1993. Patient-Mix Differences Among Ambulatory Care Providers and Their Effects on Utilization and Payments for Maryland Medicaid Users. *Medical Care, 31*(12), 1119–1137.

Thorpe, K., and Brecher, C. 1987. Improved Access to Care for the Uninsured Poor in Large Cities: Do Public Hospitals Make a Difference? *Journal of Health Politics, Policy and Law, 12*(2), 313–324.

U.S. General Accounting Office. 1996. *Rural Health Clinics: Rising Program Expenditures Not Focused on Improving Care in Isolated Areas.* Washington, DC: U.S. General Accounting Office.

Weissman, J., Dryfoos, P., and London, K. 1999. Income Levels of Bad-Debt and Free-Care Patients in Massachusetts Hospitals. *Health Affairs, 18*(4), 156–166.

West, D. 1999. Medicaid Managed Care: Linking Success to Safety-Net Provider Recruitment and Retention. *Journal of Ambulatory Care Management, 22*(4), 28–32.

Wyatt, S., Moy, E., Levin, R., Lawton, K., Witter, D., Valente, E., Lala, R., and Griner, P. 1997. Patients Transferred to Academic Medical Centers and Other Hospitals: Characteristics, Resource Use, and Outcomes. *Academic Medicine, 72*(10), 921–930.

Zuvekas, A., McNamara, K., and Bernstein, C. 1999. Measuring the Primary Care Experiences of Low-Income and Minority Patients. *Journal of Ambulatory Care Management, 22*(4), 63–78.

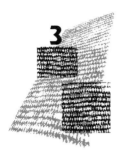

Forces Affecting Safety Net Providers in a Changing Health Care Environment

Several recent studies have warned that changes in the health care marketplace may threaten the ability of safety net providers to continue serving the poor and uninsured (Altman et al., 1998; Andrulis, 1997; Baxter and Mechanic, 1997; Fishman and Bentley, 1997; Lipson and Naierman, 1996; Norton and Lipson, 1998). To date, safety net providers have demonstrated considerable resiliency in maintaining their missions of caring for uninsured and other vulnerable populations. Recent changes within the health care marketplace, however, threaten to intensify pressures on safety net providers. This chapter provides a detailed examination of the many forces affecting safety net providers' fiscal viability and their ability to care for uninsured and other vulnerable populations.

There are major and increasing variations in states' capacities and willingness to support care for vulnerable populations. The organization, financing, and adequacy of the health care safety net varies substantially from state to state and from community to community. In the absence of federally sponsored universal insurance coverage, care for uninsured and other vulnerable populations is increasingly influenced by state and local policies. The wide variation in the structures and the conditions of the safety nets across states, however, make national tracking and comparative analysis in this area difficult.

The sources and intensities of the pressures facing individual providers depend on the level of demand, amount of support, and the structure of the safety net in a community. The structural characteristics of the safety net and the factors that affect safety net providers are illustrated in Figure 3.1.

The horizontal continuum of Figure 3.1 depicts the major structural factors that influence local safety net systems. Essential factors that determine the structure of local safety nets include

- The degree of formal or informal organization of the safety net,
- The extent to which care for Medicaid beneficiaries and uninsured individuals is concentrated among a few providers or shared among many,
- The degree to which the safety net system is comprised of public or private entities,
- The level of price competition, and
- The extent of Medicaid managed care penetration.

The safety net system itself can be formal in its organization, relying on horizontal or vertical networks, public authorities, or other defined governance structures, or it can be informal, relying on the actions of individual providers to cover care for uninsured and other vulnerable

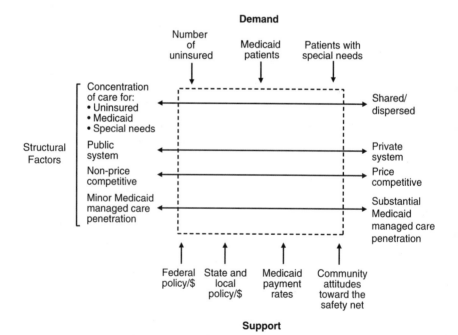

FIGURE 3.1 Factors affecting the health care safety net.

populations. In some communities one or two publicly subsidized providers, such as a large public hospital or a hospital partnered with a well-defined network of community health centers (CHCs), may be responsible for nearly all of the health care for the uninsured population. In other communities health care for uninsured individuals might be widely dispersed among many providers, including not-for-profit providers and other mission-driven hospitals. Highly concentrated safety net systems tend to rely on public providers and tight organizational structures, whereas widely dispersed systems are more likely to comprise a mix of public and private providers and rely on less formal organizational structures. The level of price competition in a community and the degree of Medicaid managed care penetration can also significantly shape local safety net systems and influence their stability.

Safety net systems are neither uniform nor static; that is, no single paradigm describes them perfectly and no single approach will sustain them. Moreover, it is important to understand the structural aspects of each safety net to predict the effects of major forces of change on its future viability. The paragraphs below offer three examples of different safety net structures, those in Miami, Florida; Philadelphia, Pennsylvania; and Boston, Massachusetts.

Miami's safety net is an example of a moderately concentrated, formally organized public safety net in a community with large numbers of uninsured people. Dade County, where Miami is located, is a highly competitive, mature managed care market for both commercial and Medicaid businesses (Lipson et al., 1997). Jackson Memorial Hospital, a public teaching hospital, is the major provider of care for vulnerable populations. It not only provides services at its own locations but also is responsible for operating the clinics of the local health department. Health care for indigent populations in Miami as well as in many other parts of the state is supported primarily by local taxing districts. Jackson Memorial Hospital has recently reached out to a larger community of providers by affiliating with CHCs and other hospitals, although there are still some safety net providers that are not part of the Jackson Memorial Hospital network.

On the other end of the continuum is Philadelphia, a city with large uninsured and Medicaid populations but without a publicly owned hospital since 1978. With the closing of Philadelphia General, the city's nine public health stations were converted to community-based primary care programs. The health department clinics, along with six federally qualified health centers (FQHCs), have been participating in some form of managed care since the mid-1980s. Philadelphia's inpatient safety net is informally organized and is dispersed among several academic health centers and other public and private hospitals. Philadelphia has an active health care market that offers some degree of choice to vulnerable populations and high-price competition. As a result, the safety net comprises multiple competing networks, each of which provides some care to the safety net population (National Health Policy Forum, 1998).

Boston is a market with significant managed care penetration. Prompted by state Medicaid policies, Boston has an array of small and large, public and private not-for-profit organizations that work together to craft the local safety net. In this configuration, the treatment of vulnerable populations is dispersed among CHCs, private not-for-profit providers, and the public hospital systems organized into relatively formal networks. CHCs have formed networks, have sponsored health plans, and have entered into multiple affiliations to strengthen their ability to serve the indigent population. Concurrently, Boston City Hospital merged with Boston University Medical Center to create the Boston Medical Center with the expectation that an integrated organization would be better able to provide continued services to vulnerable populations. Local health center networks have linked with the medical center to provide a cohesive, integrated system of care for vulnerable populations. To support these efforts, organizations can receive funds from a pool of funds for state-sponsored health care for the indigent population (Baxter and Feldman, 1999).

These examples provide only snapshots of very complicated safety net systems. They are intended simply to illustrate the local variability of safety net systems. Although virtually all local safety net systems rely on a core group of providers for either ambulatory care, inpatient care, or both, no single structural configuration of the safety net is right for all communities. It is clear, however, that the way in which a local safety net is structured will have a lot to do with how it adapts to the major forces of change described in the remainder of this chapter.

The primary challenges that currently affect safety net providers can be grouped into three areas: (1) increasing demand for care by uninsured and other vulnerable populations, (2) uncertain public support (federal, state, and local) for safety net providers, and (3) the changing structure and environment of the broader health care system and the resulting disequilibrium caused by changes in the payer mix. This chapter examines each of these forces in detail.

INCREASING DEMAND FOR CARE

The increasing demand for safety net care can be traced to several phenomena, including trends in the number of uninsured individuals (including the length of time that they remain without coverage and the geographic variation in the number of uninsured people across the country), the number of underinsured Americans, the impact of welfare

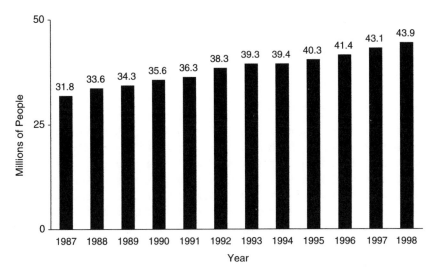

FIGURE 3.2 Number of uninsured nonelderly Americans (in millions), 1987 to 1998. Medicaid and uninsured data from 1998 are not completely consistent with previous years. Starting with the March 1998 Current Population Survey (CPS), the Bureau of the Census modified its definition of the population with Medicaid and the population without health insurance. Previously, individuals covered solely by the Indian Health Service were counted in the Medicaid population. Beginning with data from the 1998 CPS, individuals covered solely by the Indian Health Service are counted as uninsured. SOURCE: Fronstin (2000). Reprinted with permission of the Employee Benefit Research Institute.

reform, and the limited success of recent efforts to expand insurance coverage.

Trends in the Number of Uninsured

The level of demand for safety net care is driven most directly by the sheer number of persons without health insurance in the local area. Despite the overall strength of the U.S. economy, the number of uninsured nonelderly Americans increased by 30 percent between 1988 and 1998, from 33.6 million to 43.9 million (Figure 3.2). During that time, the percentage of uninsured Americans rose from 15.5 to 18.4 percent of the nonelderly population.[1] Nearly all the increase between 1996 and 1998, from 17.7 to 18.4 percent, was accounted for by adults ages 18 to 64.

---

[1]These figures represent the most recent data available, which are from the March 1998 Supplement of the Current Population Survey (CPS) (Fronstin, 2000).

Several factors contributed to the growing number of uninsured individuals in the United States and thus the increased demand for free services faced by safety net providers. These are delineated in the following sections.

Decline in Employer-Sponsored Coverage

The proportion of nonelderly Americans receiving health insurance through their employers declined 4.1 percent between 1988 and 1998, with the greatest declines being among low-income workers and families. More than 83 percent of those without insurance in 1998 lived in families headed by workers (Fronstin, 2000). The proportion of nonelderly employees who receive their health insurance from employers declined sharply from 69.2 percent in 1987 to a low of 63.5 percent in 1993, but it then increased to 64.2 percent in 1997, according to the Census Bureau. Slightly more employers are offering health insurance, but fewer workers are taking it either because the employee's portion of the coverage is too costly or because of a lack of eligibility due to waiting periods or number of hours worked. However, the largest number of uninsured are salaried workers whose employers do not sponsor health insurance.[2]

Exacerbating the erosion of employer-based coverage is the rapid growth of part-time, contract, and temporary jobs that typically offer no benefits. In 1997, 29 percent of the U.S. workforce held "nonstandard" jobs that were temporary, part-time, contract, or day-labor positions (Mishel et al., 1998). Figure 3.3 shows that over the last decade the percentage of low-wage workers who had access to employer-sponsored insurance through their own job or that of a family member decreased. Even greater declines occurred in the percentage of low-wage workers who had access to insurance and were actually covered by it (i.e., family take-up rate).

Workers with incomes of between 100 and 200 percent of the federal poverty level,[3] often referred to as the "near poor," are especially vulnerable. Caught between ineligibility for Medicaid and inadequate resources

---

[2]Virtually all large employers offer health insurance coverage to their full-time workers, although only 60 percent of small businesses do so. The most recent 1999 Annual Employer Health Benefits Survey found little change in the number of plans that offer health insurance coverage over the last 2 years (Kaiser Family Foundation/Health Research and Educational Trust, 1999).

[3]The federal poverty level in 1997 for a family of three with two adults and one child was $12,919 and for a family of three with one adult with two children was $12,931; 300 percent of the poverty level is the equivalent of $39,000. The median family income in 1997 for a family of three was $46,783 (Dalaker and Naifeh, 1998).

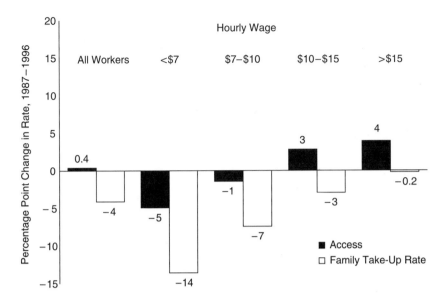

FIGURE 3.3 Employers offering health insurance and worker participation, 1987 to 1996, by wage of workers. SOURCE: O'Brien et al. (1999). Calculations based on data from Cooper and Schone (1997). Reprinted with permission of the Institute of Health Care Research and Policy.

to buy their own insurance, the near poor run the highest risk of being uninsured. In 1997 a third of individuals in families with incomes less than 200 percent of the federal poverty level were uninsured, whereas just 9 percent of those with family incomes above 300 percent of the federal poverty level were uninsured (O'Brien et al., 1999). It is precisely these low-income uninsured families who most often rely on safety net providers for their health care. The rising number of uninsured individuals at a time when unemployment rates are approaching a 30-year low does not bode well for the future unless there is a dramatic change in national policy (Kuttner, 1998). The demand for uncompensated care and the need for safety net services in this environment promise to increase and accelerate.

Decline in Public Coverage

Since 1993, increases in the number of uninsured individuals have been driven by declines in public coverage (Fronstin, 1999). Although Medicaid covers many low-income families who meet program eligibility requirements, a large number of eligible families do not gain access to

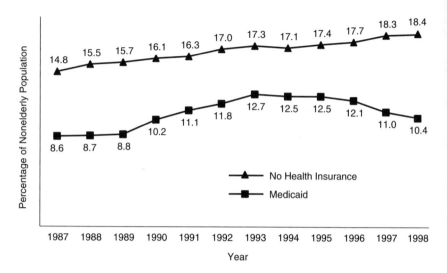

FIGURE 3.4 Trends in Medicaid coverage and a lack of health insurance coverage, 1987 to 1998. Medicaid and uninsured data from 1998 are not completely consistent with previous years. Starting with the March 1998 Current Population Survey, the Bureau of the Census modified its definition of the population with Medicaid and the population without health insurance. Previously, individuals covered solely by the Indian Health Service were counted in the Medicaid population. Beginning with data from the 1998 CPS, individuals covered solely by the Indian Health Service are counted as uninsured. SOURCE: Fronstin (2000). Reprinted with permission of the Employee Benefit Research Institute.

coverage. In 1998 less than half (44.8 percent) of nonelderly Americans with family incomes below the federal poverty level were covered by publicly sponsored health insurance.[4] Declines in public coverage are especially important to safety net providers since publicly insured individuals make up a large proportion of safety net providers' paying patient base. Declines in public coverage are apt to have a large effect on safety net providers' bottom line. Figure 3.4 illustrates the changing trends in Medicaid coverage and the number of uninsured individuals from 1987 to 1998.

---

[4]According to March 1999 CPS data, 41.6 percent of nonelderly respondents with family incomes below the federal poverty level were insured by Medicaid, with the remaining 3.2 percent accounted for by other sources of public coverage, including Medicare, the Civilian Health and Medical Program of the Uniformed Services, the Civilian Health and Medical Program of the Veterans Administration, and U.S. Department of Veteran's Affairs health insurance (Fronstin, 2000).

Growth in Length of Time Without Insurance

The demand for uncompensated care from safety net providers also is affected by the length of time that uninsured individuals remain without coverage. Point-in-time estimates or "snapshots" of the number of uninsured, such as those generated by the Current Population Survey (CPS), must be placed in context. If the average length of time that each uninsured person remains without coverage grows, overall demand for uncompensated care can also be expected to grow. An analysis of the 1994–1995 Survey of Income and Program Participation data found that approximately half of all spells without health insurance lasted for 8 months or longer,[5] and about a third of all uninsured individuals are uncovered for the entire year (Copeland, 1998). This subgroup of chronically uninsured individuals is especially likely to depend on safety net providers for health care.

Geographic Variation in the Number of Uninsured

Although national trends are clearly troubling, it is the distribution of uninsured families across states and local communities that most directly determines the pressure that individual safety net providers will face. As seen in Figure 3.5, uninsured Americans are heavily concentrated in the southwestern and south-central states. In 12 states,[6] more than 20 percent of the population is uninsured (Fronstin, 2000).

The variation in the concentration of uninsured individuals is more dramatic when comparing different metropolitan areas. According to the March 1999 CPS data, the Houston, Texas, metropolitan area had the highest percentage of uninsured nonelderly residents in 1998, with more than 30 percent, followed by Los Angeles, California, with more than 29 percent and Miami, Florida, with 25 percent (Fronstin, 2000). Safety net providers in these metropolitan areas are likely to face much greater demand for uncompensated care than those safety net providers located in areas with fewer uninsured individuals. Several factors explain such variation. Perhaps most importantly, immigrant populations—both legal and illegal immigrants—are highly concentrated in a handful of states. Three states (California, New York, and Texas) account for 64 percent of the estimated 5 million undocumented immigrants and 57 percent of the

---

[5]The median spell of 8 months is longer than that reported in earlier studies by Bennefield (1996) and Swartz et al. (1993), which found the median spell without insurance to be approximately 6 months.

[6]Arizona, Texas, California, New Mexico, Nevada, Mississippi, Montana, Arkansas, Louisiana, Oklahoma, Florida, and West Virginia.

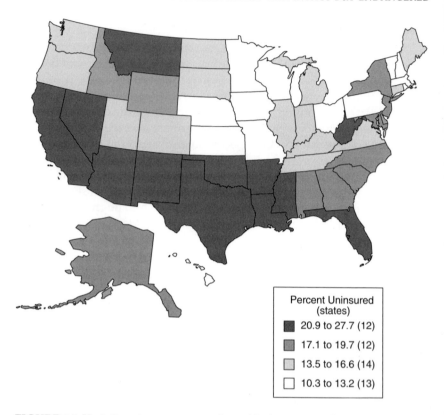

FIGURE 3.5 Variations in percentage of nonelderly uninsured among U.S. states and the District of Columbia, 1998. SOURCE: Unpublished calculations by A. Shields based on Current Population Survey data presented in Fronstin (2000). Reprinted with permission of the Institute of Health Care Research and Policy.

legal immigrants in the United States.[7] Changes enacted in the Personal Responsibility and Work Opportunity Reconciliation Act (PRWORA; P.L. 104–193) of 1996, discussed in greater detail below, have increased the number of legal immigrants who are ineligible for publicly sponsored health insurance. Safety net providers in states with large immigrant populations will thus experience greater demand for uncompensated care than providers in other states.

---

[7]These states account for only 26 percent of the total U.S. population (U.S. Bureau of the Census, 1999). Calculations by A. Shields, Institute for Health Care Research and Policy, Georgetown University, based on Immigration and Naturalization Service estimates as of April 1996 (see Immigration and Naturalization Service, 2000a; Immigration and Naturalization Service, 2000b).

The number of uninsured individuals and the demand for free care are also directly affected by individual states' Medicaid eligibility rules, the breadth and depth of their Medicaid benefits packages, and their payment rates. In states with meager benefits packages, safety net providers may provide free services to individuals who have Medicaid coverage but who need services not included in the benefits package. Lastly, the relative wealth and the tax base of each state vary greatly. A study by Marquis and Long (1997) showed serious geographic disparity between the distribution of uninsured individuals and the distribution of the ability to finance subsidized health insurance for them. States with the largest number of uninsured people, which would be required to tax their residents more heavily to have a significant impact on the problem, are precisely the states with lower income bases to begin with (Marquis and Long, 1997).

Underinsurance

Demand for uncompensated care comes not only from uninsured individuals but also from those whose insurance is inadequate to cover the costs of their health care needs. As many as one of every eight families (12 percent) without elderly members spent, on average, more than 10 percent of the family income on out-of-pocket health care costs and premium cost-sharing in 1997; families with members over age 65 spent 50 percent of the family income on health-related costs (Shearer, 1998). An earlier study found 18.5 percent of the U.S. population to be underinsured in 1994 (Short and Banthin, 1995). Depending on the definition of underinsurance that one uses, between 10 and 25 percent of those with health insurance have inadequate coverage to protect them against financial risk. In times of medical crisis, many of these individuals are unable to pay for uncovered services and must rely on safety net providers for free care. The committee also read and heard evidence during its workshops and deliberations suggesting that rising drug costs are leading many uninsured and low-income insured individuals to seek care from safety net providers where drugs may be free or heavily subsidized. Findings from a 1997 United Hospital Fund survey on the access of uninsured individuals to outpatient services in New York City showed that 74 percent of public hospitals, 39 percent of financially distressed hospitals, and 47 percent of FQHCs provided discounts on drugs, whereas 8 percent of voluntary hospitals provided such discounts (United Hospital Fund, 1998).

The Impact of Welfare Reform

After a period of steadily increasing Medicaid enrollment that began in the late 1980s, Medicaid enrollment has declined steadily since 1995. Although much of this decline can be attributed to a robust economy, reduced Medicaid enrollment has been exacerbated by the impact of welfare reform. The PRWORA (P.L. 104–193), also known as the "welfare reform law," was enacted in August 1996.[8] This legislation was intended to reduce the number of families who receive cash assistance and to encourage work participation,[9] but it may have had secondary consequences for the Medicaid program. Welfare reform severed the link between welfare and Medicaid eligibility, essentially "delinking" cash assistance and Medicaid coverage. Before the enactment of PRWORA, any person who received Aid to Families with Dependent Children (AFDC) was automatically eligible for Medicaid coverage. Despite efforts to preserve the independence of Medicaid eligibility from welfare assistance, there have been widespread difficulties in doing so, resulting in marked reductions in Medicaid enrollments (Ellwood and Ku, 1998; Maloy et al., 1998; Smith et al., 1998). State programs designed to divert families from cash assistance also appear to be impeding many eligible families from being enrolled in Medicaid (Maloy et al., 1998).

The PRWORA also includes provisions that cause many legal immigrants to become ineligible for Medicaid coverage. According to the statute, legal immigrants who entered the United States after August 22, 1996, are ineligible for Medicaid for the first 5 years that they live in the United States, with few exceptions (Sections 402 and 403, P.L.104–193). After the initial 5-year bar, it is up to each state to decide whether to offer Medicaid eligibility.[10] This law also affects access to the new State Children's Health Insurance Program (SCHIP). Immigrant children who arrived after August 22, 1996, are ineligible for SCHIP for the first 5 years that they are in the country; after that time, however, their eligibility is mandatory. Although 18 states have initiated some form of state-

---

[8]PRWORA ended the individual entitlement to welfare benefits under Aid to Families with Dependent Children (AFDC), which had been established by the Social Security Act of 1935.

[9]Officials from the U.S. Department of Health and Human Services recently noted that the last several years have produced the "largest caseload decline in history," with welfare rolls falling from an all-time high of 14.3 million in January 1994 to an estimated 8.9 million in March 1998 (State Health Notes, 1998).

[10]Medicaid eligibility for immigrants entering the United States prior to August 22, 1996, is also each state's option, although for this group, all states except Wyoming have extended Medicaid eligibility to immigrants who arrived in the United States before August 22, 1996 (Carmody, 1998). Examples of immigrant groups exempted from the 5-year ban include refugees and those who have been granted political asylum.

sponsored medical assistance to legal immigrants affected by the new law, only about half provide assistance to all groups of legal immigrants who lost their eligibility for Medicaid (Carmody, 1998).

These changes in immigration law have led to widespread confusion. Recent studies report that many eligible immigrants are reluctant to apply for Medicaid because they believe they are ineligible or worry that applying may adversely affect their immigration status or chances of attaining citizenship (Ellwood and Ku, 1998). In addition to eliminating eligibility for Medicaid, other changes in public support for recent immigrants, such as the curtailment of food stamp benefits, may also affect the ability of low-income uninsured immigrants to pay for needed health care.

To the extent that states fail to address the widespread confusion that has kept many Medicaid-eligible persons from applying for Medicaid, safety net providers will face greater pressure to provide care for un-insured individuals. In a recent survey by the National Association of Community Health Centers (1998), CHC directors ranked welfare reform as the number one issue negatively affecting their paying patient base. Persons who delay enrollment in Medicaid and who remain uninsured may also have greater health care needs than those of the traditional Medicaid population in the past. If there is a significant change in the case mix of the Medicaid population over time and if Medicaid capitation rates are not adjusted accordingly, financial pressures on safety net providers will further intensify.

Although the full impact of welfare reform on Medicaid enrollment has not yet been determined, the most recent available data indicate significant decreases in enrollment among the nonelderly Medicaid population. Between 1995 and 1998, the percentage of nonelderly Americans enrolled in Medicaid fell from 12.5 percent to 10.4 percent, a 16.8 percent reduction. The number of Medicaid beneficiaries receiving cash assistance fell by 13 percent for adults and 11 percent for children in 1997, despite expansions in coverage for children (The Kaiser Commission on Medicaid and the Uninsured, 1999). Figure 3.6 shows trends in the rate of Medicaid enrollment by eligibility group for the period from 1990 to 1997.

Limited Success of Incremental Efforts to Expand Coverage

Medicaid Waivers

Several state and federal initiatives to expand health insurance coverage have had various degrees of success. Many states have used the mechanism of Health Care Financing Administration (HCFA) Section 1115 demonstration waivers to expand Medicaid coverage to groups that otherwise would not have met the Medicaid eligibility criteria. These waivers

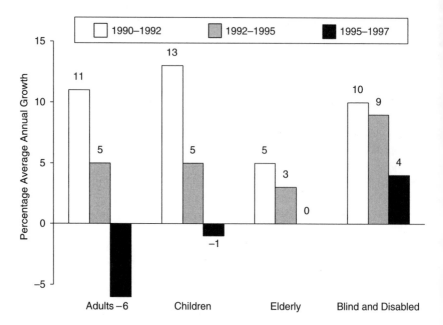

FIGURE 3.6 Rate of growth in Medicaid enrollment by eligibility group, 1990 to 1997. SOURCE: The Kaiser Commission on Medicaid and the Uninsured (1999). Reprinted with permission.

also allow states to collect federal matching funds for the costs of coverage or services for such groups, which otherwise would not be available. As of April 1999, 17 states have implemented Section 1115 waivers.[11]

Recent state-specific evidence shows some increase in access for previously uninsured populations through Section 1115 waivers. However, most of the gains in coverage were realized in the initial years of the state initiatives, and the numbers of individuals gaining access have fallen short of original expectations (Hoag et al., 1999; Kalkines, Arky, Zall and Bernstein, LLP, 1999).

Both Oregon and Tennessee have reduced the number of uninsured individuals in the state (Aizer et al., 1999; Mittler et al.,1999). In Tennessee, for example, the proportion of the state population that is uninsured declined from 8.9 percent in 1993 to 5.9 percent in 1997, which translates

---

[11]Alabama, Arizona, Arkansas, Delaware, Hawaii, Kentucky, Maryland, Massachusetts, Minnesota, Missouri, New York, Ohio, Oklahoma, Oregon, Rhode Island, Tennessee, and Vermont.

into 130,000 newly insured individuals under the state TennCare program (Aizer et al., 1999). Medicaid enrollment in Oregon has stagnated in recent years, with a decline since 1994 in both newly eligible individuals and individuals who have traditionally been eligible for Medicaid (MDS Associates, 1999). TennCare's enrollment in January 1998 was 1.2 million, reflecting no real gains since 1994 (MDS Associates, 1999).

Even in states where gains in coverage have been achieved, they have not been sufficient to reduce the demand for safety net care noticeably. In a five-state study, safety net providers reported that the demand for uncompensated and subsidized care had not decreased even in locations where state initiatives had successfully expanded coverage (Gold et al., 1996). The demand for services had been greater than the supply; thus, improved access to care for the newly covered comes at the expense of access to care for those who remain uninsured (Gold et al., 1996).

Figure 3.7 lists the percentage changes in Medicaid enrollment from 1995 to 1997. Contrary to national trends, 10 states increased their Medicaid enrollments either through their waiver programs, or, in the case of New Mexico, New Hampshire, Nebraska, Washington, and Alaska, through eligibility expansions and significant outreach efforts (U.S. General Accounting Office, 1999).

Health Insurance Portability and Accountability Act

The Health Insurance Portability and Accountability Act of 1996 (HIPAA; P.L. 104–191) included provisions that had the potential to provide some help to those with insurance to help prevent them from losing coverage. HIPAA's narrow legal focus, however, prevented it from doing much to expand coverage. The Act limits the use of preexisting condition exclusion clauses to deny coverage and guarantees the availability and renewability of health insurance. But HIPAA fails to address the issue of affordability by allowing insurers to price their policies as they see fit (some states have, however, established rating bans). The Act also includes provisions for a medical savings accounts (MSAs) demonstration project for up to 750,000 people and gradually increases tax deductions related to health insurance premiums for self-employed individuals from 30 percent in 1996 to 80 percent by 2006 (Wilensky, 1998). At best, these provisions might result in expanded rates of coverage among the higher-income working uninsured.[12]

---

[12]According to Internal Revenue Service reports (Internal Revenue Service, 1998), as of June 1998 only 54,702 taxpayers had established MSAs, and over 17,000 of these had previously been insured (Fronstin, 1998).

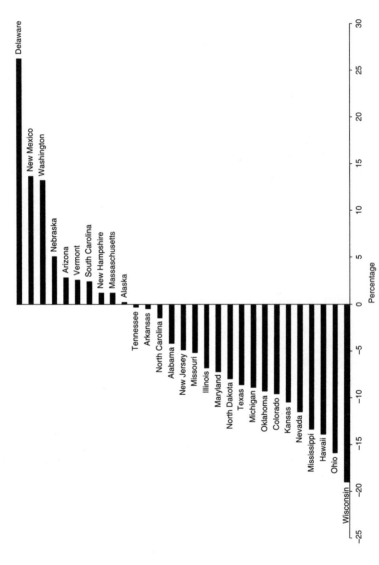

FIGURE 3.7 Percentage changes in selected states' Medicaid enrollment, 1995 to 1997. SOURCE: U.S. General Accounting Office (1999).

State Children's Health Insurance Program

A more recent program, SCHIP, which is Title XXI of the Balanced Budget Act (BBA) of 1997 (P.L. 105–33), may hold more promise. SCHIP is a federal grant-in-aid program that offers states support for programs aimed at providing "child health assistance" to "targeted low-income children." Its goal is to reduce the number of uninsured children while providing states with maximum flexibility. SCHIP will provide states $20.3 billion between 1998 and 2002 and nearly $19.4 billion over the second 5 years. It includes specific provisions to bar SCHIP from supplanting the existing Medicaid effort and addresses concerns about the crowding out of private insurance by limiting SCHIP coverage to children without other forms of "creditable coverage"[13] (Rosenbaum et al., 1998).

The Congressional Budget Office (CBO) initially projected that SCHIP would cover 2.8 million previously uninsured children,[14] with another 600,000 children enrolled in Medicaid through SCHIP outreach and eligibility screening (Rosenbaum et al., 1998). All states with the exceptions of Wyoming, Washington, and the District of Columbia, have developed or are in the process of developing a SCHIP implementation plan.[15]

The major problem with SCHIP, however, has been difficulty in enrolling eligible children. States have experienced substantial delays in the implementation of SCHIP, and most jurisdictions are already falling significantly behind their initial enrollment schedules. SCHIP faces the same challenges of identifying and enrolling eligible children that the Medicaid program faces. It is estimated that as many as 4.7 million children are potentially eligible for Medicaid coverage but are not yet enrolled (Selden et al., 1999). As of December 1998, 40 states (including the District of Columbia) had together enrolled only 834,790 children in SCHIP. Enrollment efforts in recent months have been more successful. SCHIP enroll-

---

[13]The term "creditable coverage," as defined in HIPAA (P.L. 104–191), includes health insurance, employer health plans, Medicaid, and other public or private third-party assistance (Rosenbaum et al., 1998).

[14]The actual number of children finally enrolled will depend on the level of outreach, ease of access, and cost-sharing requirements. A recent Kaiser Commission report estimates that between 79 and 83 percent of uninsured children whose family's incomes are below 200 percent of the federal poverty level will participate if SCHIP coverage is free and easy to obtain. This figure drops to a range of 24 to 38 percent with the addition of a modest premium of only $17 per month or $200 per year (The Kaiser Commission on Medicaid and the Uninsured, 1998a).

[15]States have considerable latitude in designing their programs. Twenty states are opting to expand their Medicaid programs, 14 are developing new programs that subsidize private insurance, and 15 are combining the two approaches (Reschovsky and Cunningham, 1998).

ment increased 57 percent during the 6 month period spanning December 1998 to June 1999, from 834,790 to 1,310,959 children (Smith, 1999).[16]

Even if these positive trends continue, this major expansion of public insurance is expected to reach only about a third of all uninsured children. Given that children as a group have relatively inexpensive health care needs, it is not likely that SCHIP will do much to reduce the demand for uncompensated care from safety net providers.

UNCERTAINTIES IN PUBLIC SUPPORT

Disproportionate Share Hospital Payments

An important source of federal support for safety net hospitals is Medicaid disproportionate share hospital (DSH) payments. Since the early 1990s, Medicaid DSH payments have supported hospital-based care for uninsured patients, and safety net hospitals have become particularly dependent on the DSH program.[17] In 1997, Medicaid DSH payments to hospitals totaled nearly $16 billion (Congressional Budget Office, 1998).[18]

As seen in Figure 3.8, Medicaid DSH payments exploded in the early 1990s, and although they have declined in recent years, they still remain a significant source of funding for hospitals. The Omnibus Budget Reconciliation Act of 1996 included provisions that allowed states to pay hospitals that serve large numbers of low-income patients more than Medicare rates (thus exceeding the "Medicare upper payment limit"[19]), and earlier HCFA rulings in 1985 allowed states to receive donations from providers. These two changes led to an explosion in expenditures on DSH payments

---

[16]SCHIP may also help increase the number of Medicaid-eligible children who actually gain Medicaid coverage. According to a recent national survey of SCHIP, many states report finding one or more Medicaid-eligible children for every SCHIP enrollee (Smith, 1999).

[17]States are required to make additional payments to hospitals that served a disproportionate share of low-income and Medicaid patients, although not for the uninsured per se. These hospitals are known as disproportionate share hospitals. DSH payments are made to hospitals that have Medicaid utilization rates more than one standard deviation above the mean Medicaid utilization rate for participating hospitals in their state or a utilization rate by low-income individuals of greater than 25 percent. States may also treat as a disproportionate share hospital any facility, including state mental hospitals, with an inpatient Medicaid utilization rate of greater than 1 percent (Rosenbaum and Darnell, 1997).

[18]Medicare DSH payments also are important to many hospitals, although they represent a much smaller source of revenue, approximately $4.5 billion in 1997, compared with nearly $16 billion in Medicaid DSH payments in the same year (Congressional Budget Office, 1998).

[19]The "Medicare upper payment limit" refers to a regulation passed by HCFA in 1983 stating that states could not pay more in the aggregate for Medicaid inpatient care or long-term-care services than what would have been paid under the Medicare program.

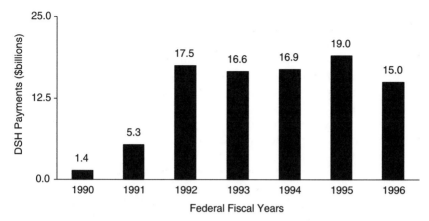

FIGURE 3.8 Medicaid spending on DSH payments, 1990 to 1996. SOURCE: Coughlin and Liska (1997) based on data from HCFA 64 Forms. Reprinted with permission of The Urban Institute.

in the early 1990s, from $1.4 billion in 1990 to $17.5 billion by 1992 (Coughlin and Liska, 1997). States quickly learned how to use the DSH payment program to generate federal dollars by substituting provider taxes, provider donations, or intergovernmental transfers for the state share of "expenditures" to justify their receipt of federal "matching" dollars.[20] The state contribution for DSH payments often is a contribution on paper only as states maneuver to garner federal dollars with minimal state outlays.[21]

As a result of these changes, money available for DSH payments is shrinking. The BBA of 1997 further reduces federal DSH payments[22] to

---

[20]A typical scenario might look like this one, offered by Coughlin and Liska (1997): A state receives a $10 million tax or donation from a provider. The state then makes a $12 million payment back to the same provider, either in a lump-sum payment or through increased rates, which represents a $2 million gain for the provider. If the state's federal matching rate is 50 percent (they range from 50 to 80 percent), the state would be reimbursed for half of the $12 million payment by the federal government. In this scenario, the state receives $6 million from the federal government, but only $2 million of this actually goes to the provider that serves low-income patients. The remainder is kept by the state for other purposes.

[21]A recent study of DSH payments in 13 states (that together represent 60 percent of national expenditures on DSH payments) found that most states rely exclusively on intergovernmental transfers for state financing, but some relied heavily on health-related taxes and a few relied on state general revenue (Coughlin and Liska, 1998).

[22]The BBA of 1997 also stipulates that DSH payments can no longer be incorporated into the capitated rate to managed care organizations, as a number of states had done. For example, four states included DSH payments in their capitation rates under risk-based managed care programs in 1998 (Holahan et al., 1999).

states by $10.4 billion from fiscal year 1998 to 2002 (Congressional Budget Office, 1997), with actual payment levels set forth for each state for each fiscal year through 2002.[23] The Urban Institute has estimated that the BBA of 1997 related reductions in federal spending on DSH payments from 1998 to 2002 relative to actual spending on DSH payments in 1995 represent an 11 percent decrease in federal spending on DSH payments (Coughlin and Liska, 1998).

The DSH payment program is not particularly effective in targeting public resources to providers who serve uninsured patients. A recent study reported, for example, that DSH payments per Medicaid or uninsured person in each state ranged from less than $1 per person in several states to nearly $700 in Connecticut (Coughlin et al., 2000).

Aside from recent reductions in funding for DSH payments, several other factors mitigate against the effectiveness of the DSH payment program as a mechanism to finance care for uninsured individuals. First, the pressures of increased competition have caused many nontraditional safety net providers to seek Medicaid patients as a source of revenue, which then allows them to seek funding through DSH payments. As Medicaid patients are channeled into managed care, safety net hospitals are losing Medicaid patients and DSH payment revenues. The current formula allows providers to qualify for DSH payments on the basis of their Medicaid volume alone and does not require an explicit level of commitment to the uninsured population. The Medicare Payment Advisory Commission recently recommended changes in the DSH payment allocation formula that will assess a provider's volume of uninsured patients separately from its Medicaid case load, although the formula has yet to be modified (Medicare Payment Advisory Commission, 1999).

Second, the hospital focus of the DSH payment program excludes non-hospital providers. In some instances, local hospital systems allow CHCs or other ambulatory care providers to receive DSH payments, although these funds are typically restricted to hospital-based providers. This is at odds with the general trend toward outpatient care and managed care, which emphasizes primary care and preventive services. It also leaves community-based ambulatory care clinics, which often have the most meager financial reserves, with no comparable source of support.

Lastly, a substantial portion of DSH payments never reaches the hospitals that provide care for the uninsured population or even the hospitals that serve Medicaid patients; instead, they are retained by state officials

---

[23]After 2002, DSH payments for each state will rise by an amount equal to the medical care component of the Consumer Price Index for urban consumers, with aggregate DSH payments capped at 12 percent of a state's total Medicaid expenditures (Rosenbaum and Darnell, 1997).

for other purposes. A 1993 survey of 39 states found that one-third of DSH payments were retained by states and were not paid to disproportionate share hospitals (Ku and Coughlin, 1995), although more recent data indicate that a greater proportion of DSH payments have reached providers in recent years (Coughlin et al., 2000). Comparisons of data from a 1993 survey of disproportionate share hospitals with data from a 1997 survey showed that in 1997 hospitals netted about 60 percent of total revenues available through the DSH payment program, up from 35 percent in 1993 (Coughlin et al., 2000).

Recent Federal Medicaid Policy Changes

In addition to the DSH payment provisions described above, the BBA of 1997 (P.L.105–33) makes many significant changes in the structure of Medicaid eligibility, the use of managed care, provider reimbursement, and long-term care. CBO has estimated that these changes will result in a total of $13 billion in savings in Medicaid spending over 5 years, including the $10.4 billion reduction in Medicaid DSH payments discussed above. Policy changes contained in the BBA of 1997 have significant implications for both ambulatory care and hospital-based providers. Some of the key provisions[24] are discussed below.

Phaseout of Cost-Based Medicaid Reimbursement

The BBA phased out cost-based Medicaid reimbursement for FQHCs by the year 2003. Under the provisions, states were to reimburse FQHCs 100 percent of reasonable costs during fiscal years 1998 and 1999. The phaseout of Medicaid cost-based reimbursement for FQHCs was to begin with a 5 percent reduction in fiscal year 2000. Allowable reductions then progressed to 10 percent in fiscal year 2001, 15 percent in 2002, and 30 percent in 2003 (Rosenbaum and Darnell, 1997).

The Balanced Budget Refinements Act (BBA 1999 P.L.106–113), passed on November 29, 1999, delays the implementation of a 10 percent reduction in cost-based reimbursement to 2003, with a 15 percent reduction implemented in fiscal year 2003 (Table 3.1). This new legislation also requires that GAO conduct a comprehensive study before 2001 to assess the impact of these reductions on FQHCs and the populations they serve before any further reductions are instituted. Under these provisions, as was the case with the BBA, states can opt to continue cost-based reim-

---

[24]For an exhaustive review of the Medicaid-related provisions in the BBA of 1997, see Rosenbaum and Darnell (1997). For additional analysis of the financial provisions and the assumptions on which they were based, see Schneider (1997).

TABLE 3.1 Changes in the Balanced Budget Act (BBA) of 1997 Phaseout of Health Center Cost-Based Reimbursement Made by the BBA Refinements Act of 1999

Act	Percentage in Fiscal Year							
	1999	2000	2001	2002	2003	2004	2005	2006
1997 BBA	100	95	90	85	70	50	50	50
1999 BBA Refinements	100	95	95	95	90	85	50	50
Difference	0	0	5	10	20	35	0	0

SOURCE: National Association of Community Health Centers (1999b). Reprinted with permission.

bursement if they wish. A March 1999 survey conducted by the National Association of Community Health Centers found that at least 24 states plan to continue paying FQHCs under cost-based reimbursement (National Association of Community Health Centers, 1999a.)[25] Although this recent legislation goes a long way toward shoring up FQHCs' financial stability in the short run, the long term financial stability of FQHCs is not secure and may depend on the level of support individual FQHCs are able to command at the state and local level.

Prior to the establishment of the FQHC Program in 1989, some state Medicaid agencies were paying the centers far below the costs of basic medical care—in some cases as low as $9 to $10 per visit. Thus, federal grants that were intended to fund care for uninsured patients and special non-medical services were actually subsidizing the Medicaid program. As a result, cost-based reimbursement was instituted as part of the establishment of the Medicare and Medicaid Federally Qualified Health Centers Program to recognize the reasonable costs of caring for Medicaid patients. Legislation established cost-based reimbursement for organizations that receive grants through the Bureau of Primary Health Care (i.e., community health centers, migrant health centers, health care for the homeless programs, and public housing primary care programs), for Native American outpatient clinics, and for other health centers that are designated as FQHC "look-alikes."[26] These centers were to be paid a cost-related per-visit rate. The method of setting this rate varied among states

---

[25]Six states have already introduced legislation to this effect, while the remaining 18 states anticipate using some combination of administrative or budget mechanisms to effectively maintain cost-based reimbursement for CHCs.

[26]CHCs certified as FQHC "look-alikes" are CHCs that meet federal grant standards but that do not actually receive federal grants.

and many but not all states adopted caps and screens similar to those prescribed for Medicare FQHC payments. Some implemented the program within a few years, others were much slower.

Receiving the full cost for services provided to Medicaid patients allowed FQHCs to expand their service capacity and achieve a marginal degree of financial stability. Cost-based reimbursement covered the costs of organizational infrastructure and staffing and thus allowed FQHCs to serve many more patients, both insured and uninsured. The phaseout of cost-based reimbursement greatly increases the fiscal vulnerability of these programs, which together serve over 10 million patients. (For details on the population served, see Chapter 2.)

Provisions Related to Medicaid Managed Care

The federal government affects funding for safety net providers not only directly through reimbursement policies but also indirectly through policy changes that bear on safety net providers' access to patients. The BBA of 1997 allows states to implement mandatory Medicaid managed care programs without the need for Section 1915(b) (demonstration) waivers and diminishes the need for Section 1115 (research and demonstration) waivers for some groups (excluding individuals with dual eligibility, i.e., those eligible for both Medicare and Medicaid, children with special health care needs, children in foster care, and Native Americans) (Rosenbaum and Darnell, 1997). State initiatives under the new provisions likely will increase the dispersion of Medicaid patients throughout the health care delivery system, thus reducing the number of Medicaid patients and revenues available to safety net providers.

Local Support for Inpatient Safety Net Providers

Safety net providers are often dependent on state and local government support to remain fiscally solvent. Crises in supporting care for uninsured and other vulnerable populations are often resolved at the local level. The relative importance of state support, over and above DSH payments, versus the importance of local support to safety net hospitals varies greatly. Some states specifically assign responsibility for care for indigent populations to counties. These funds typically represent 5 to 10 percent of the total budgets of safety net hospitals. In some locations, such as Harris County (Houston, Texas) and Dade County (Miami, Florida), public hospitals receive an exceptionally high level of funding from the county, whereas in others support is more limited. The level of local support received by safety net providers depends in no small degree on the political will of the community, its attitudes toward vulnerable popu-

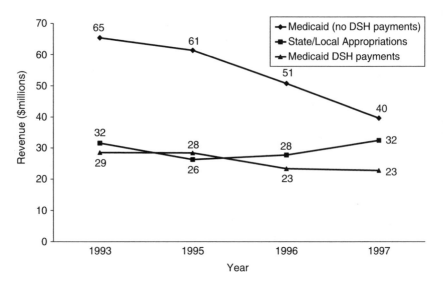

FIGURE 3.9 Average net revenues from select sources at NAPH member hospitals, 1993 to 1997. Analysis includes data from 33 of 68 NAPH member hospitals for which complete data were available. *t* tests indicate no significant difference in average revenues between hospitals with complete time series and those with incomplete time series. SOURCE: Unpublished analysis of American Hospital Association Annual Survey Data, 1990 and 1996 by J. Tolbert, National Association of Public Hospitals and Health Systems. Reprinted with permission of the National Association of Hospitals and Health Systems.

lations, and its attitudes toward the providers who serve them. Overall, local support for public hospitals has increased slightly since 1993, but it has not risen sufficiently to offset the losses due to the decline in Medicaid patients and the DSH payments that support their care. (Figure 3.9 illustrates these trends for a national sample of public hospitals that are members of the National Association of Public Hospitals [NAPH].[27]) State and local subsidies as a percentage of total hospital revenues among the same sample fell 6 percent between 1991 and 1997; uncompensated care as a percentage of total costs increased 3 percent over the same period (Figure 3.10).

Few studies have addressed county-level support for safety net providers, largely because of the difficulty in obtaining reliable data. One

---

[27]These figures represent data for approximately half of all NAPH member hospital systems, and include data for those hospitals for which complete data were available for all years analyzed.

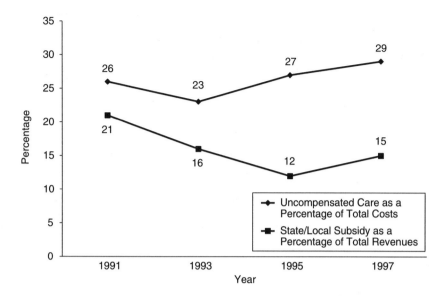

FIGURE 3.10 Trends in state and local subsidies and uncompensated care costs at NAPH member hospitals, 1991 to 1997. Analysis includes data from 37 of 68 NAPH member hospitals. t tests indicate no significant differences between hospitals with complete time series and those with incomplete time series. SOURCE: Unpublished analysis of NAPH Hospital Characteristics Survey Data, 1993–1997 by J. Tolbert, National Association of Public Hospitals and Health Systems. Reprinted with permission of the National Association of Public Hospitals and Health Systems.

recent study examined county-level efforts to fund care for the indigent population in three large urban areas: Harris County (Houston, Texas), Alameda County (Oakland, California), and Dade County (Miami, Florida). It focused particularly on the scope and stability of public subsidies to safety net hospitals (Meyer et al., 1999). At two of the three locations, safety net hospitals were running operating deficits, leaving them vulnerable to fiscal difficulty in the event of an economic downturn. For example, the principal source of funding for Jackson Memorial Hospital in Miami is a local sales tax, which would be greatly affected by a recession. Meyer and colleagues (1999) conclude that although safety net hospitals are "bumping along" so far, they are not well positioned for an uncertain future. Their success will be determined in large measure by the political skills of their leaders in coaxing local authorities to make up the revenue shortfalls (Meyer et al., 1999).

Direct and Indirect Subsidies for Graduate Medical Education

Direct and indirect subsidies for graduate medical education (GME) represent a fairly small revenue stream for safety net hospitals, approximately 10 percent of all Medicare revenues. Through GME, Medicare directly subsidizes residency programs at hospitals. Most teaching hospitals have become reliant on medical residents as an important source of medical staffing. Before the enactment of the BBA of 1997, there were no caps on levels of support for GME. The provisions of the BBA of 1997, however, impose significant reductions in funding for GME. A recent industry analysis of hospitals in New York City estimates that reductions of support for GME will result in an average 13 percent reduction in Medicare revenues and a 4 percent reduction in hospitals' bottom line, representing an average annual loss of $520 million (Wang, 1999). The new provisions in the BBA of 1997 will have a greater impact on urban safety net hospitals, which rely heavily on residents to provide patient care.

CHANGING STRUCTURE AND ENVIRONMENT OF THE HEALTH CARE MARKETPLACE

Increasing demand for uncompensated care and decreasing and uncertain revenues from federal, state, and local sources must be examined within the larger context of the rapidly changing health care marketplace. Perhaps no single factor has led to more dramatic changes in the environment for safety net providers than the overarching shift toward greater price competition. Pressure to reduce health care costs has come from both the public and private sectors and has spurred a massive restructuring of the health care system. According to a recent Urban Institute study of safety net providers in 13 states, the level of competition that they face is driven by three factors: the penetration of private managed care, the concentration of market share among providers, and the presence of for-profit providers (Norton and Lipson, 1998).

Managed Care Penetration

A recent InterStudy analysis of 322 regional markets found that in July 1998, 71.9 million Americans were enrolled in managed care plans,[28] an increase of 5.2 million from 1997 (InterStudy, 1998, 1999). Enrollment grew mainly in large metropolitan areas. The number of metropolitan

---

[28]These figures refer to health maintenance (HMO) and point-of-service (POS) plans only, and so do not include preferred provider organizations (PPOs).

areas with managed care penetration rates of at least 25 percent more than doubled from 1996 to 1998, expanding from 88 market areas in 1996 to 145 market areas in 1998 (InterStudy, 1997, 1999).

Increased rates of managed care penetration are accompanied by increased competition for patients. Reuter and Gaskin (1997), for example, found that academic medical centers in areas with high health maintenance organization (HMO) enrollments[29] experienced a decline in admissions of 10.5 percent between 1991 and 1994, whereas hospitals in areas with low HMO enrollment experienced a 0.6 percent increase in hospital admissions. Studies have also documented a relationship between increased HMO penetration and decreased levels of uncompensated care[30] (Mann et al., 1997; Thorpe et al., 1998).

Medicaid Managed Care

Increasing penetration of managed care in the Medicaid market is especially important for safety net providers, which depend on Medicaid revenues for financial stability. In recent years, public-sector officials have often used their purchasing power to ratchet down payments to providers and implement new managed care models for Medicaid beneficiaries. By June 1996, more than 25 percent of the Medicaid populations in 36 states and the District of Columbia were enrolled in managed care plans (The Kaiser Commission on the Future of Medicaid, 1997). By June 1998, 54 percent (16.6 million) of all Medicaid beneficiaries were enrolled in some form of managed care plan (Health Care Financing Administration, 1999), with all states except Alaska and Wyoming now pursuing some managed care initiative.

Managed care can offer the potential to improve patient care and coordination, expand provider accountability, and control costs. For most safety net providers, especially those in urban areas, Medicaid managed

---

[29]This study uses HMO enrollment data only, and does not include PPOs and other types of managed care entities.

[30]Although the present study focuses on core safety net providers, it should be noted that physicians as a group represent a significant source of care for the uninsured population. Managed care has also been associated with decreased provision of charity care or with care provided by physicians. A survey of 10,881 physicians in 60 randomly selected communities found, for instance, that physicians who derive at least 85 percent of their practice revenues from managed care were significantly less likely to provide charity care to uninsured patients, and when they did, they provided considerably less care to uninsured patients than physicians with little involvement in managed care (Cunningham et al., 1999). This pattern held even for physicians who practice in areas with high rates of enrollment in managed care plans, regardless of their own level of involvement with managed care.

care has also brought new and increasing competition for Medicaid patients, reduced patient census and revenue streams, complex contractual relationships, and new administrative requirements. Three central concerns confront many safety net providers with respect to Medicaid managed care: loss of Medicaid patients to other providers, the adequacy of Medicaid payment rates, and the impact of reduced Medicaid patient revenues on their ability to provide care to the increasing number of low-income uninsured people.

Loss of Medicaid Patients

To remain financially viable, safety net providers must successfully maintain (and grow) their Medicaid patient bases. Safety net providers compete in the managed care environment to various extents. Some have successfully maintained their Medicaid market share through participation in provider-sponsored managed care organizations (MCOs) or other strategies. Many safety net providers are losing some portion of their Medicaid patients, primarily as a result of declining Medicaid enrollment and, in some cases, increased competition for these patients among providers, many of whom are new to the Medicaid market. Between 1995 and 1998, for example, Medicaid patients as a proportion of all patients served by FQHCs declined from 39 to 33 percent, with the largest decrease occurring between 1995 and 1996 (see Table 3.5).

Medicaid managed care has been viewed by many Medicaid administrators as a vehicle for providing Medicaid beneficiaries a wider range of choice regarding where they receive their health care, including the opportunity to enroll in the same health plans that serve privately insured individuals. Although the goal of expanded choice is generally viewed positively, in practice the rapid and large-scale movement of large numbers of Medicaid enrollees within the health care delivery system has risks for both patients and safety net providers. For patients, there is the risk of reduced continuity of care. Some state policies do not take into account the discontinuous nature of Medicaid coverage, with patients moving back and forth between periods of Medicaid coverage and being uninsured.[31] Such circumstances seriously undermine continuity of care since there is no assurance that the Medicaid managed care provider will continue to provide care when the patient becomes uninsured. Accordingly, these patients may return to their original safety net provider for free or subsidized care once they have lost coverage. This dynamic leaves

---

[31]A recent study of Medicaid enrollment in nine states, for example, found unstable plan enrollment due to fluctuating Medicaid eligibility (Maloy and Pavetti, 1998).

safety net providers with a greater demand to provide free care and a simultaneous loss of Medicaid reimbursement during periods when their patients are eligible for Medicaid and are served elsewhere.

The extent to which safety net providers have lost Medicaid patients differs across states. Many states have responded to sharp decreases in Medicaid enrollments among safety net providers by developing default enrollment policies that favor assignment of new Medicaid enrollees to plans that use safety net providers or that have developed other initiatives aimed at helping safety net providers.

Although increased competition for Medicaid patients has had some positive effects, such as stimulating safety net providers to improve their productivity and better respond to patient demands (e.g., expanding their hours of operation and reducing their waiting times), the net loss of Medicaid patients experienced by safety net providers can undermine their financial viability. Lower Medicaid revenues make it difficult to provide care for the uninsured (on a marginal cost basis) and can also result in cutbacks in patient outreach and other enabling programs particularly associated with safety net providers.

Medicaid Rate Adequacy

The effort to expand choice for Medicaid beneficiaries through commercial managed care plans has had only limited success and has highlighted concerns about the adequacy of Medicaid rates. After dramatic early increases in rate of entry of commercial plans into the Medicaid market, many have subsequently withdrawn, often citing inadequate premium rates (Langreth, 1998). Although many plans enjoyed positive margins in the initial years of Medicaid managed care because of generous rates and favorable selection, Medicaid providers have experienced significant rate reductions in recent years. The subsequent losses experienced by plans have been at least in part responsible for the sharp decrease in the number of HMOs that participate in Medicaid. Figure 3.11 shows recent trends in HMO profits.

The emergence of Medicaid-only plans, many of which consist of traditional safety net providers, may offer new opportunities for safety net providers that are able to deliver quality care and that can effectively manage risk-based contracts. Yet, they are now left to survive on capitated rates set well below those that they received in the pre-managed care era, resulting in less revenue for the same patient populations that they previously served.

The adequacy of Medicaid capitated rates has emerged as a major concern. States currently use a variety of actuarial methodologies and procedures to develop Medicaid managed care capitated rates, as docu-

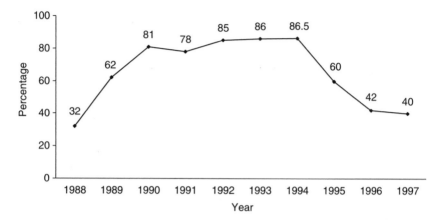

FIGURE 3.11 Percentage of HMOs reporting a profit, 1988 to 1997. SOURCE: Hurley and McCue (1998). Reprinted with permission of the Center for Health Care Strategies.

mented in a thorough review of the practices in 15 states (Schwalberg, 1997). A HCFA regulation (42 CFR 447.361) imposes an upper limit on capitation rates under risk-based contracts, stipulating that rates must not exceed the cost of providing services covered by the contract on a fee-for-service basis to an actuarially equivalent nonenrolled population group (Schneider, 1997). In future years, the lack of fee-for-service data for states that enroll most of their Medicaid beneficiaries in MCOs (which often do not provide encounter-level data) will make it even more difficult to assess rate adequacy.

The rates that providers receive under Medicaid managed care vary greatly depending on the state in which the providers are located. A recent study of Medicaid managed care rates found as much as a twofold variation in rates across states for similar populations (Holahan et al., 1999). Higher rates are associated with states whose Medicaid managed care beneficiaries are concentrated in urban rather than rural areas or with states that set higher initial rates to attract new managed care plans to the Medicaid market. On the other hand, states that carve out special populations from managed care arrangements or that provide generous DSH payment support to hospitals are more likely to set lower capitation rates. The study suggests that, in general, states that view managed care as a way to improve access for the Medicaid population are more likely to have higher capitation rates, whereas states that have historically limited fee-for-service costs through narrow benefit packages or low provider rates offer lower capitation rates.

Rate adequacy must also be considered in light of the mix of patients served. States are using various approaches to set capitation rates. Their capacity to adjust payments according to risk, however, remains rudimentary. Maryland, Massachusetts, Colorado, Washington, and Oregon have or are developing more sophisticated rate-adjustment methodologies, but most states have very little capacity to construct patient mix-adjusted Medicaid managed care. Both Maryland and Colorado use risk adjustment and risk assessment. Colorado and Oregon rely on a disability payment system that identifies and groups diagnoses that are chronic in nature and are associated with higher future costs and pays providers accordingly. Maryland classifies individuals into unique morbidity groups on the basis of their age, sex, and previous medical claims.

In the absence of adequate risk adjustment, selection bias is a particular concern. Some safety net providers claim that certain MCOs serve only healthier patients, leaving them with the sicker, more costly Medicaid patients. At least one study of children with asthma enrolled in the Massachusetts Medicaid program supports such claims (Shields, 1998). Children with a greater number of major pediatric comorbidities were 50 percent more likely to be enrolled with a traditional Medicaid provider than with the staff model HMO under study. A recent study of the 12 MCOs participating in TennCare, Tennessee's Medicaid managed care plan, found that academic health centers served Medicaid patients with a greater burden of illness (e.g., AIDS, coagulation defects, transplantation, or cystic fibrosis) than the burden of illness of Medicaid patients served by other participating MCOs (Bailey et al., 1999).

The adequacy of Medicaid payment rates relative to the health care needs of the patient populations served warrants ongoing study. Knowledge regarding how best to adjust for differences in patient populations served (and the data to do it with) remains limited, however. The danger exists that in their attempts to survive on low Medicaid rates, safety net providers will discontinue or compromise the very services that make them unique providers for special subpopulations of patients.

Impact on Safety Net Care

The growth of Medicaid managed care directly affects safety net providers' ability to maintain their safety net role. Managed care plans aim to provide quality health care services to their enrolled populations for a competitive price. Uninsured individuals do not easily fit into this framework; they are not part of the enrolled population, and the costs associated with them rarely are factored into competitive bids. In areas where intense market competition has caused other non-core safety net providers to reduce their level of effort in caring for uninsured patients, safety net providers will experience a greater demand from uninsured patients who were previously served by other community providers. Many safety net providers testifying before the committee reported that increased numbers of uninsured patients were requesting care from them as the number of Medicaid beneficiaries in managed care increased in their area.

In cases in which these reduced Medicaid revenues and the increasing demand for uncompensated care are accompanied by other reductions in federal, state, and local funding for care for indigent populations, the financial viability of safety net providers can quickly become tenuous. Although neither Medicaid programs nor managed care providers are responsible for subsidizing care for uninsured patients, the fact remains that increased competition and reduced revenues have lessened safety net providers' ability to support care for the uninsured population. Although this is not necessarily the responsibility of Medicaid administrators, it remains a public policy concern. The weakening of the safety net will reduce standby assistance for those who remain uninsured and will ultimately reduce access to an appropriate array of medical and social services for Medicaid clients if these safety net clinics are forced to close.

Conversions, Consolidation, and Concentration of Market Share

The health care market has also been marked by rapid consolidation, network expansions, conversions to for-profit status, and extensive deal-making as each provider group or organization scrambles to ensure its market share and financial viability. Most research on conversions and their impact on care for vulnerable populations has focused on the hospital sector (Claxton et al., 1998; Gray, 1998; Needleman et al., 1997; Reuter and Gaskin, 1998). Among a national sample of 5,768 hospitals, more than 12 percent of hospitals changed ownership status between 1980 and 1993, with more than half of these occurring in Alabama, California, Florida, Georgia, Missouri, and Texas. The extent of conversions can also be measured by looking at the number of hospital beds affected. Between 1981 and 1995, the proportion of community hospital beds accounted for by for-profit entities grew from 9 to 12 percent. The proportion of for-profit hospitals as a percentage of all community hospitals increased from 13 to 14 percent over the same period (The Kaiser Commission on Medicaid and the Uninsured, 1998b).

Public hospitals around the country have affiliated with or have been acquired by private hospitals or hospital systems at a rapid rate in recent years (Legnini et al., 1999).[32] From 1985 to 1995, the number of public hospitals declined by 14 percent (Legnini et al., 1999). In a major study conducted for The Commonwealth Fund, some conversions of public hospitals to private ownership were described by hospital representatives as an effort to improve efficiency by freeing the public hospitals from civil service and procurement rules. More often, however, they were described as a response to the unwillingness of local governments and communities to provide continued tax support for these hospitals (Needleman et al., 1997).

Findings from a Henry J. Kaiser Foundation study of privatization of public hospitals indicates that in most instances, after conversion, access to care for low-income patients is preserved and teaching programs have not been cut (Legnini et al., 1999). Respondents to the Kaiser Foundation study highlighted that the access issue would require continued monitoring by the community. Another recent study on the issue provides a different perspective, however. An analysis of uncompensated care and hospital conversions in Florida between 1981 and 1996 showed that after conversion, uncompensated care declined significantly among public hospitals. These hospitals had demonstrated a significant commitment to supporting charity care before the conversion (Needleman et al., 1999). In contrast, nonprofit hospitals showed little change in their levels of uncompensated care following conversion to for-profit ownership. It is important to note, however, that these converting hospitals delivered less uncompensated care before conversion than non-converting hospitals of the same type. This suggests that for many nonprofit hospitals, conversion to for-profit status may not have a significant negative impact on the provision of uncompensated care in the community because it may represent the last stage in a process of reducing a hospital's safety net role in an effort to cope with financial losses (Needleman et al., 1999).

Health plans are also converting from nonprofit to for-profit status. The increased corporate influence in health care is especially evident in the growing prevalence of for-profit companies within the HMO sector. Between 1981 and 1997, the for-profit HMO representation of total HMO enrollees grew from 12 to 62 percent, and for-profit HMO representation grew from 18 to 75 percent over the same period (The Kaiser Commission on Medicaid and the Uninsured, 1998b).

Financial Disequilibrium

The general trend of decreased Medicaid revenues and increased

---

[32]Public hospitals (other than those run by the federal government) account for almost one-quarter of the community hospitals in the United States.

numbers of uninsured has left many safety net providers in a financially precarious position. Some have been more successful than others in maintaining or even increasing their Medicaid revenues in the competitive Medicaid managed care market, whereas others have experienced tumultuous revenue losses. Hospitals, CHCs, and local health departments (LHDs) have all experienced this disequilibrium to a certain extent, although the largest effects thus far have been found among certain subgroups of providers.

Hospitals

Comparisons of the financial performances of different types of hospitals in 1992 and 1997 are shown in Tables 3.2 and 3.3.[33] Overall, hospitals did quite well in these 6 years. Net gains for community hospitals grew from 4.8 percent in 1992 to 7.2 percent in 1997. The main reason for the overall financial improvement of hospitals was the growth in payments relative to costs associated with Medicare patients. In 1992, Medicare payments were substantially below costs at –4.4 percent. By 1997, payments relative to costs had risen to a net gain of 1.4 percent. Medicaid also showed some improvement. In contrast, the favorable position of private patient revenues deteriorated from a net gain of 11.8 percent to one of 6.7 percent. It is higher payments from the latter patients that usually provide hospitals with the margins to provide care for those without health insurance coverage. Care for those who did not pay all or a portion of their bill (uncompensated care) grew from a loss of –4.9 percent to one of –5.2 percent.

The declining financial conditions of public major teaching hospitals are noteworthy. The positive gains for this group of hospitals fell from 2.8 to 1.6 percent between 1992 and 1997. The American Hospital Association (AHA) considers positive margins under 2 percent as breaking even and a sign of serious financial trouble (National Health Policy Forum, 1999). The significance of this decline is that it occurred during a period when the overall financial performance of hospitals in general almost doubled. A major reason for the decline in the financial health of these safety net institutions was the increase in losses from uncompensated care, which rose from –7.3 percent in 1992 to –10.2 percent in 1997.

Core safety net hospitals are losing patients in selected areas where they previously realized healthy margins, such as low-risk maternity care. A recent study by Gaskin and colleagues (2001) present evidence that

---

[33]Although these tables use the same data sources (American Hospital Association Annual Survey of Hospitals), the hospital groupings are slightly different because the tables were developed at different times.

from 1991 to 1994 the markets for Medicaid maternity patients became more competitive, whereas the care for uninsured maternity patients became more concentrated in safety net hospitals (Figure 3.12). Safety net hospitals in large metropolitan statistical areas in California, Florida, Massachusetts, and New Jersey lost their market shares of Medicaid maternity patients, whereas they gained larger shares of uninsured maternity patients. New York was the only state in that study in which safety net hospitals increased their share of Medicaid maternity patients. This was probably due to New York's hospital rate-setting system, which shields hospitals from price competition caused by managed care.

For core safety net providers such as public hospitals, the trend of increasing numbers of uninsured individuals and decreasing numbers of Medicaid patients is more dramatic. Figure 3.13 illustrates the trends among a national sample of 39 public hospitals that experienced an average 12 percentage-point decline in the proportion of Medicaid discharges in recent years, from 57 percent in 1993 to 45 percent in 1997. Over the same period, these hospitals saw a 6 point increase in the percentage of self-paying patients, most of whom are uninsured. It is not clear what proportion of the decline in Medicaid admissions is due to recent declines

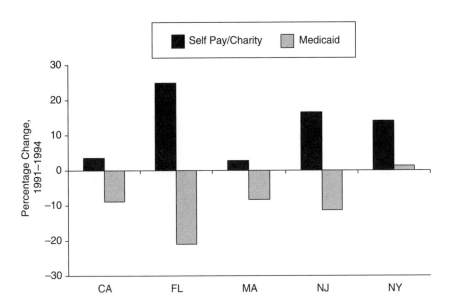

FIGURE 3.12 Change in safety net hospitals' market shares of Medicaid and uninsured patients, 1991 to 1994. SOURCE: Gaskin et al. (2001). Reprinted with permission of the Institute for Health Care Research and Policy.

TABLE 3.2 Hospital Gains and Losses by Payer, by Hospital Group, 1992

Hospital Group	Gains or Losses as a Percentage of Total Cost					
	Medicare[a]	Medicaid	Uncompensated Care[b]	Private	All Others[c]	Aggregate Total Gain
All community hospitals	-4.4	-1.2	-4.9	11.8	3.5	4.8
Public major teaching	-1.2	1.5	-7.3	5.6	4.2	2.8
Nonpublic major teaching	-2.9	-1.3	-4.8	8.6	4.1	3.6
Other teaching	-4.5	-1.0	-4.9	12.0	3.5	5.1
Nonteaching	-5.4	-1.6	-4.6	13.9	3.1	5.3
Voluntary	-4.4	-1.5	-4.6	11.6	3.6	4.7
Proprietary	-6.2	-2.1	-3.9	17.4	1.1	6.3
Urban government	-2.8	0.9	-6.9	8.8	4.3	4.3
Rural government	-4.4	-0.2	-5.0	11.5	4.2	6.1

NOTE: Owing to reporting inconsistencies related to Medicaid DSH payments and provider-specific taxes, there are significant margins of error for the numbers related to all payers in 1992.

[a]Medicare and Medicaid costs equal all costs; both inpatient and outpatient, attributed by hospitals to these programs' patients regardless of whether the costs are allowable (and therefore reimbursable) by the programs.

[b]Operating subsidies from state and local governments were considered payments for uncompensated care up to the level of each hospital's uncompensated care costs. Additional subsidies above this level were counted as corporate revenue.

[c]Includes other government health programs and nonpatient businesses.

SOURCE: Medicare Payment Advisory Commission analysis of data from the American Hospital Association Annual Survey of Hospitals.

TABLE 3.3 Hospital Gains and Losses by Payer, by Hospital Group, 1997

Hospital Group	Gains or Losses as a Percentage of Total Cost					
	Medicare	Medicaid	Uncompensated Care	Private	All Others[a]	Total
All community hospitals	1.4	-0.5	-5.2	6.7	4.8	7.2
Public major teaching	2.5	1.3	-10.2	9.2	-1.2	1.6
Private major teaching	1.3	-1.6	-5.2	4.0	6.4	4.8
Other teaching						
Public other teaching	1.2	0.4	-9.3	9.7	4.1	6.1
Private other teaching	0.6	-0.9	-4.7	7.9	5.4	8.3
Nonteaching						
Public nonteaching	-1.6	-1.5	-4.7	10.5	4.8	7.6
Private nonteaching	0.3	-1.3	-4.5	10.1	4.5	9.2
Voluntary	0.4	-1.4	-4.7	7.3	5.7	7.3
Proprietary	5.1	-0.1	-4.5	13.3	2.0	15.6
Urban government	1.8	0.5	-9.0	8.2	2.1	3.7
Rural government	-2.4	-1.2	-4.4	11.0	5.0	8.0

NOTES: Gains or losses are the difference between the cost of providing care and the payment received. Operating subsidies from state and local governments are considered payment for uncompensated care, up to the level of each hospital's uncompensated care costs. Data are for community hospitals and reflect both inpatient and outpatient services. Most Medicare and Medicaid managed care patients are included in the private payers' category. U.S. totals were calculated using reported and imputed data; values for groups reflect reported data only.

[a]Includes other government health programs and nonpatient business.

SOURCE: Medicare Payment Advisory Commission analysis of data from the American Hospital Association Annual Survey of Hospitals.

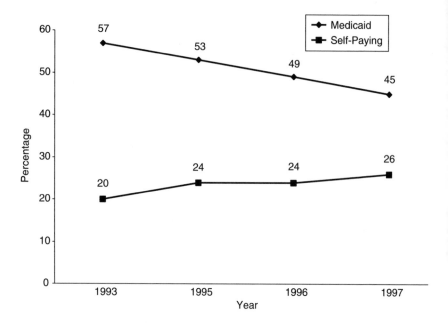

FIGURE 3.13 Medicaid and self-paying patient discharges as a percentage of total discharges at NAPH member hospitals, 1993 to 1997. The analysis includes data from 39 of 68 NAPH member hospitals. *t* tests indicate no significant difference in total discharges between hospitals with complete time series and those with incomplete time series. SOURCE: Unpublished analysis of NAPH Hospital Characteristics Survey data, 1993–1997, by J. Tolbert, National Association of Public Hospitals and Health Systems. Reprinted with permission of the National Association of Public Hospitals and Health Systems.

in the number of persons who receive Medicaid and what proportion is due to the dispersion of these patients to non-safety net providers.

This increasing concentration of uncompensated care patients in safety net hospitals was reported by many hospital administrators in public forums conducted by IOM as part of this study. Safety net providers testified that the confluence of Medicaid managed care, increased price competition, decreased federal and local support, and increased numbers of uninsured individuals has led to a greater concentration of uninsured patients at their hospitals and a simultaneous dispersion of Medicaid patients and revenues to non-safety net hospitals.

The committee also heard several witnesses express concern that the overall financial conditions of hospitals committed to providing care for poor and uninsured populations will deteriorate further with fuller impact

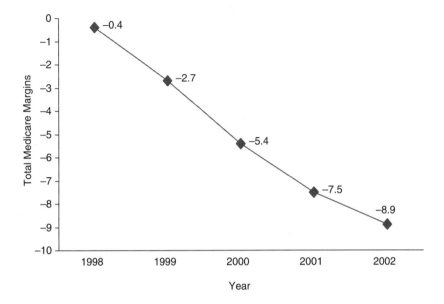

FIGURE 3.14 Actual and projected declines of total Medicare margins for public hospitals as a result of the BBA of 1997. Data include impatient preferred provider services (PPS), home health PPS, and PPS-exempt. SOURCE: Unpublished analysis of Medicare cost report data by The Lewin Group. Reprinted with permission of The Lewin Group.

of the BBA of 1997. Medicare margins, which had been rising through 1997, are projected to decline. This decline in margins is expected to make even more precarious the financial positions of public as well as other mission-driven hospitals (Figure 3.14).

Community Health Centers

For CHCs, the decade of the 1990s has been characterized by two trends. First, the centers became much more dependent on Medicaid, leaving them more vulnerable than ever to changes in the marketplace. Second, the number of uninsured patients has continued to grow, potentially forcing hard choices between the CHCs' mission to serve all patients and their need to survive. Analysis of CHCs source of revenues and utilization and revenues per user illustrates this dilemma.

Both the volume and the composition of revenue of FQHCs changed significantly between 1990 and 1998. As Table 3.4 indicates, total revenues grew from $1.2 to $3.1 billion during that time. Although revenues from

TABLE 3.4 Trends in Federally Qualified Health Center Revenue, 1990–1998

Revenue Source	Total Revenues (percent) (in $ millions)				
	1990	1995	1996	1997	1998
Total	$1,239 (100)	$2,465 (100)	$2,754 (100)	$2,845 (100)	$3,110 (100)
Bureau of Primary Health Care Grant	508 (41)	640 (26)	727 (26)	698 (25)	746 (24)
Other federal grants	13 (1)	56 (2)	50 (2)	68 (2)	74 (2)
Medicaid	254 (21)	816 (33)	937 (34)	985 (35)	1049 (34)
Medicare	72 (6)	157 (6)	178 (6.5)	191 (7)	201 (6.5)
Other insurance	108 (9)	208 (8)	211 (8)	253 (9)	309 (10)
Patient payments	115 (9)	165 (7)	172 (6)	183 (6)	204 (7)
State/local/other	169 (14)	422 (17)	479 (17)	466 (16)	527 (17)

SOURCE: Unpublished tabulations of Uniform Data System data by the Health Resources Services Administration, U.S. Department of Health and Human Services.

all sources increased, the growth was primarily driven by the implementation of FQHC cost-based reimbursement. Not only did Medicaid pay its fair share (as the proportion of revenues approximated the proportion of covered patients), but it fueled a major increase in the total number of patients served and a reduction in the dependence on federal grant funding. Thus Medicaid, which accounted for 21 percent of total revenues in 1990, increased to 33 percent of total revenues in 1995 and 34 percent of total revenues in 1998. Conversely federal grants accounted for 42 percent of the total revenues in 1990, 28 percent in 1990 and 26 percent in 1998. The rate of growth for all components slowed substantially in the last two years.

Table 3.5 summarizes trends in the patient mix of FQHCs for the same time period. In 1990, FQHCs served 5.84 million patients, including 2.22 million uninsured patients and 1.87 million Medicaid beneficiaries. By 1998, FQHCs' total patient base grew to 8.66 million patients, including 3.55 million uninsured patients and 2.84 million Medicaid beneficiaries. The proportion of FQHC patients with Medicaid coverage rose from 32 percent in 1990 to 39 percent in 1995, fell to 34 percent in 1996 and then to 33 percent in 1998. In contrast, the proportion of uninsured users fell from 38 to 35 percent from 1990 to 1995 and then increased to 40 percent in 1996 and to 41 percent in 1998.

Table 3.6 examines trends in revenue per user for Medicaid, uninsured, and all FQHC patients. Medicaid revenues per Medicaid user grew substantially between 1990 and 1995, from $136 to $260, reflecting the

TABLE 3.5 Trends in Federally Qualified Health Center Users, 1990–1998

Users	Number (percent) of Users (in millions)				
	1990	1995	1996	1997	1998
Total	5.84 (100)	8.05 (100)	8.09 (100)	8.25 (100)	8.66 (100)
Medicaid	1.87 (32)	3.14 (39)	2.77 (34)	2.82 (34)	2.84 (33)
Medicare	0.58 (10)	0.75 (9)	0.63 (8)	0.63 (8)	0.62 (7)
Other insurance	1.17 (20)	1.38 (17)	1.45 (18)	1.52 (18)	1.645 (19)
Uninsured	2.22 (38)	2.79 (35)	3.24 (40)	3.33 (40)	3.55 (41)

NOTES: The 1990 data are only for community and migrant health centers; the 1995 data for CHC users include an estimate for homeless patients; the data for 1996–1998 include all Bureau of Primary Health Care grantees. The 1990 and 1995 data for FQHC users by payer are from grant applications; data for 1996–1998 are from Uniform Data System reports.

SOURCE: Unpublished tabulations of Uniform Data System data by the Health Resources Services Administration, U.S. Department of Health and Human Services.

TABLE 3.6 Trends in Federally Qualified Health Center Revenues per Patient User, 1990–1998

	Revenue per User				
	1990	1995	1996	1997	1998
Total revenue/total user	$212	$306	$340	$345	$359
Medicaid revenue/Medicaid user	136	260	338	349	369
Federal grants/uninsured user	235	249	243	230	231
Noninsurance patient care revenue[a]/uninsured user	273	319	308	288	297

[a]Estimated by adding revenues from federal grants, patient payments, state/local/other sources and subtracting the portion of total revenues (15 percent) attributable to social and enabling services.

SOURCE: Calculated from data in Tables 3-1 and 3-4, Bureau of Primary Health Care, Health Resources and Services Administration, U.S. Department of Health and Human Services.

implementation of FQHC cost-based reimbursement. There was also a big jump between 1995 and 1996, from $260 to $338 in 1996, partially due to continuing FQHC implementation but also due to the 12 percent decrease in Medicaid users in that year. At this point participation in Medicaid managed care was minimal in most areas and its impact had yet to be felt. Thereafter, Medicaid revenue per Medicaid user grew slowly to $349 in 1997 and $369 in 1998.

In an effort to understand the dynamics behind these trends, MDS Associates analyzed components of Medicaid revenues for the Health Resources and Services Administration (HRSA). They found that in 14 states, FQHCs received unusually large reconciliation payments in 1998 which were attributable to multiple prior years, and thus were unlikely to be part of a past or future trend. These payments accounted for $37 million, or 10 percent of all health center Medicaid revenues in the relevant states. Excluding this sum from 1998 Medicaid revenues in all states would reduce Medicaid revenue per user to $356—only a 2 percent increase over 1997, less than an inflation adjustment (MDS Associates, 1999).

Growth in revenue per uninsured user was slower than for Medicaid in the early 1990s, slowing or in some cases reversing in more recent years. Federal grants, the major source of revenue for care for people lacking coverage, totaled $235 per uninsured user in 1990 and $249 in 1995, a scanty increase over the five-year period. Thereafter they decreased to $243 in 1996 and $230 in 1997 and rose slightly to $231 in 1998.

A more inclusive method of estimating the funds available for medical care to uninsured patients is to add all non-insurance revenue sources—federal grants, patient sliding fee payments, and state, local and other grants—and then, since these funds are also the source of social support and enabling services for all FQHC users, to subtract out the amount attributable to such services. This yields larger amounts but a pattern not dissimilar to that found for federal grants alone. Non-insurance revenues per uninsured user were $273 in 1990, rose to $319 in 1995, fell to $308 in 1996 and $288 in 1997, and rose slightly to $297 in 1998.

In sum, in the early part of the decade Medicaid and non-insurance revenues balanced each other out as components of total revenues, so that the total revenue increased from $212 per user in 1990 to $306 in 1995 and $340 in 1996. As with the components, growth in total per patient revenue has flattened in recent years, to $345 in 1997 and $359 in 1998.

Analysis of possible reasons for shifts in revenues and utilization by HRSA did not reveal consistent relationships with state variables, including changes in the number of individuals eligible for Medicaid and changes in Medicaid expenditures for ambulatory care. Some centers that lost Medicaid patients or revenues were in states where Medicaid enrollments or expenditures for ambulatory care increased, while others were in states where enrollments or expenditures decreased. However, this analysis also suggested that national and state figures might be masking more targeted distress: centers with 30 percent or more of their patients in Medicaid managed care averaged losses in Medicaid revenues per Medicaid user of 13 percent (Lewis-Idema and Bryant, 1998). Revenue losses are

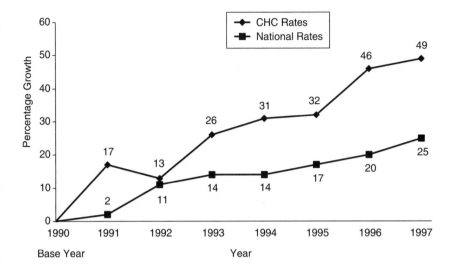

FIGURE 3.15 Percentage growth in numbers of uninsured compared with 1990 levels: rates for CHCs versus national rates. SOURCE: Health Resources and Services Administration calculations based on Current Population Survey and Bureau of Primary Health Care Annual Reporting Systems for 1990 and 1997.

likely to become more prevalent as managed care participation grows and FQHC protections are phased out.

The ability of CHCs to succeed in future years is directly related to their ability to respond to the increasing number of uninsured patients that they serve in a more competitive, demanding environment. The number of uninsured patients served by FQHCs has grown at nearly double the rate of the number of uninsured persons in the general population since 1990 (see Figure 3.15). In addition, there is evidence that a significant proportion of the new uninsured patients had previously used other providers who were now demanding payments they could not make (Lefkowitz and Todd, 1999). The rising number of uninsured patients in the absence of revenue streams to support such care could threaten the fiscal viability of CHCs.

Local Health Departments

Since most LHDs do not provide the full range of services and hours of operation typically specified in managed care contracts, their safety net role has been affected by Medicaid managed care. As Medicaid managed care has become more widespread, it has been more difficult for LHDs to participate in the Medicaid market and thus garner Medicaid revenues to offset the costs of caring for uninsured patients. In many instances, LHDs lack the required infrastructure, such as 24-hour coverage or provision of the full range of primary care services, needed to secure Medicaid managed care contracts. Although some LHDs have been successful in contracting with Medicaid HMOs, many more have encountered barriers to inclusion in managed care networks.

The inability of some health departments to respond to these requirements combined with a preexisting trend to focus on population-based public health activities has led many health departments to reduce or eliminate direct health care services. The extent of this shift away from the direct provision of primary care services was confirmed in national survey of 413 LHDs conducted in March 1999 (Shields et al., 1999). The LHDs surveyed included all LHDs in a jurisdiction with a population of greater than 100,000 (urban LHDs) as well as a national sample of LHDs with smaller jurisdictions (nonurban LHDs). Among LHDs that were providing comprehensive primary care services in 1995, 22.9 percent of urban and 17.5 percent of nonurban[34] LHDs had stopped providing such services by 1999 (Shields et al., 1999). Although some LHDs began providing direct health care services during the period from 1995 to 1999,[35] many more curtailed such programs, particularly in the area of services for women and children. Nearly 20 percent of urban LHDs and 9.4 percent of nonurban LHDs that provided comprehensive primary care services to women in 1995 had eliminated these services by 1999. Approximately 20 percent of urban health departments and 15.5 percent of nonurban health departments had eliminated comprehensive primary care services for children over the same period. These figures most likely underestimate the net loss of services provided to Medicaid and uninsured patients since they reflect absolute curtailment only and do not capture reductions in volume.

The primary reason for the elimination of direct care services differed among urban and nonurban LHDs. For urban agencies, the decision to stop providing direct primary care services most often reflected a shift in

---

[34]Nonurban LHDs refer to those in jurisdictions with populations of less than 100,000 and include members of the National Association of City and County Health Officials (NACCHO). Urban health departments include those LHDs in jurisdictions with populations of 100,000 or more, all of which are CityMatCH members and many of which are NACCHO members (Shields et al., 1999).

[35]Some LHDs actually began providing comprehensive primary care services, particularly to women and children, during the period from 1995 to 1999, although many more eliminated such services (Shields et al., 1999).

mission and focus, with inadequate funding or inadequate Medicaid reimbursement being the second most prevalent reason offered. Inadequate funding and inadequate Medicaid reimbursement were the primary reasons cited by health departments that serve jurisdictions with less than 100,000 people (Shields et al., 1999). Few public health officers reported having mechanisms in place to track whether former clients were receiving health care services elsewhere or were going without health care as a result of the reduction or elimination of services in their areas.

In many areas, LHDs not only provide primary care but also provide other health care services that may not be readily available elsewhere. These, too, may be affected by reduced Medicaid revenues and payment rates and the increasing number of uninsured clients. Since 1995 urban LHDs reported decreases in the number of specific services provided in all areas except human immunodeficiency virus (HIV) infection and Acquired Immune Deficiency Syndrome (AIDS) treatment (Shields et al., 1999). The trend among nonurban LHDs is quite different. Between 1995 and 1999, there was a net increase in direct service programs for a number of areas, including HIV infection and AIDS treatment, sexually transmitted disease (STD) treatment, adult immunizations, family planning, substance abuse services, and dental health treatment.[36] This trend reflects the reliance on LHDs for a significant amount of direct services in areas with fewer providers.

In many instances, LHDs have not curtailed direct services altogether but rather have delegated the provision of specific services to outside organizations. A recent study of the privatization of services provided by LHDs found that 57 percent of the 380 LHDs surveyed now delegate the direct performance of at least one service that was formerly performed within the health department (Keane et al., 1999). Approximately half (52 percent) have contracted out at least one public health service from the very inception of the service. Personal health services are most commonly privatized; 67 percent of all services privatized over the last decade were some form of personal health services. The primary reasons cited for privatization were lack of capacity or expertise, cost or efficiency, low volume, and a desire to collaborate with and not compete with other providers (Keane et al., 1999). LHDs that serve the largest jurisdictions were 4.3 times more likely to privatize services than LHDs that serve the smallest jurisdictions (Keane et al., 1999).

---

[36]Interestingly, more than 40 percent of local health departments surveyed began providing direct dental services, 14.6 percent began providing HIV infection- and AIDS-related services, and 4.7 percent began offering STD treatment services since 1995 (Shields et al., 1999).

Few data are available that track trends in the volume of services provided by LHDs and the insurance status of the clients served. It is difficult, therefore, to assess the impact of Medicaid managed care and state and local support on the role of LHDs in providing safety net care. Research shows that between 1992 and 1996, the number of users of Medicaid Early Periodic Screening, Detection, and Testing services in Alabama fell 24 percent, whereas the number of users of maternity services declined by 15 percent (Wall, 1998). In Florida, health departments experienced a 19 percent reduction in clients between 1991 and 1996. In Mississippi health departments provided 57 percent of the state's prenatal care services in 1993, but this fell to less than 50 percent in 1996 following implementation of its Medicaid primary care case management plan. The extent to which these service reductions at LHDs represent a shift of volume to other providers or a net loss of safety net services to vulnerable populations in the community is unknown.

CONCLUSION

In summary, the combined forces of increasing demand for uncompensated care because of the rising number of uninsured people, uncertain revenues from federal, state and local sources, and increased price competition and managed care penetration have placed safety net providers in a highly tenuous financial position. Despite a robust economy and budget surpluses at the federal and state levels, the number of Americans without health insurance and thus the number who rely on safety net providers for their health care continues to grow. At the same time, Medicaid managed care and increased competition have more generally led to increased competition for Medicaid patients and thus have threatened Medicaid revenues for safety net providers.

The hospitals, health centers, clinics, and LHDs that continue to serve large numbers of uninsured patients are coping with fewer paying Medicaid patients and restrictions on payments for the Medicaid patients who remain. The stability and adequacy of the revenue streams that support such care are further threatened by the future impact of reduced DSH payments to hospitals, the end of cost-based reimbursement for FQHCs, and the unreliability of local support.

Despite these challenges, safety net providers have demonstrated resiliency and an ability to participate in the managed care marketplace. Few, however, have secured long-term stability, even as the number of uninsured individuals continues to rise and demand for charity care is becoming more acute. The impacts of these forces of change on the health care safety net demand close monitoring. At risk is the availability of needed medical care for the nation's 44 million people who are uninsured.

REFERENCES

Aizer, A. Gold, M., and Schoen, C. 1999. *Managed Care and Low-Income Populations: Four Years' Experience with TennCare*. Washington, DC: The Henry J. Kaiser Family Foundation.

Altman, S., Reinhardt, U., and Shields, A. (eds.). 1998. *The Future U.S. Health Care System: Who Will Care for the Poor and Uninsured*? Chicago, IL: Health Administration Press.

Andrulis, D. 1997. The Public Sector in Health Care: Evolution or Dissolution? *Health Affairs* 16(4), 131–140.

Bailey, J., Van Brunt, D., Mirvis, D., McDaniel, S., Spears, C., Chang, C., and Schaberg, D. 1999. Academic Managed Care Organizations and Adverse Selection Under Medicaid Managed Care in Tennessee. *JAMA 282*(11), 1067–1072.

Baxter, R., and Feldman, R.L. 1999. *Staying in the Game: Health System Change Challenges Care for the Poor*. Fairfax, VA: Center for Studying Health System Change.

Baxter, R., and Mechanic, R.E. 1997. The Status of Local Health Care Safety Nets. *Health Affairs, 16*(4), 7–23.

Bennefield, R.L. 1996. *Dynamics of Economic Well-Being: Health Insurance, 1992 to 1993*, pp. 70–54. In: *Current Population Reports*. U.S. Bureau of the Census. Washington, DC: U.S. Government Printing Office.

Carmody, K. 1998. *State Options to Assist Legal Immigrants Ineligible for Federal Benefits*. Washington, DC: Center on Budget and Policy Priorities.

Claxton, G., Feder, J., Shactman, D., and Altman, S. 1998. Converting from Nonprofit to For-Profit. *Health Affairs, 16*(2), 9.

Congressional Budget Office. 1997. *Budgetary Implications of the Balanced Budget Act of 1997*. Washington, DC: Congressional Budget Office.

Congressional Budget Office. 1998. *The Economic and Budget Outlook: Fiscal Years 1999–2008*. Washington, DC: Congressional Budget Office.

Cooper, P., and Schone, B. 1997. More Offers, Fewer Takers for Employment-Based Health Insurance: 1987 and 1996. *Health Affairs, 16*(6), 142–149.

Copeland, C. 1998. Characteristics of the Nonelderly with Selected Sources of Health Insurance and Lengths of Uninsured Spells. *EBRI Issue Brief, 198*, 1–26.

Coughlin, T., and Liska, D. 1997. *The Medicaid Disproportionate Share Hospital Payment Program: Background and Issues*. New Federalism Issues and Options for States, Series A, No. A-14. Washington, DC: The Urban Institute.

Coughlin, T., and Liska, D. 1998. Changing State and Federal Payment Policies for Medicaid Disproportionate Share Hospitals. *Health Affairs, 17*(3), 118–135.

Coughlin, T., Ku, L., and Kim, J. 2000. *Reforming the Medicaid Disproportionate Share Program in the 1990s*. Washington, DC: The Urban Institute.

Cunningham, P., Grossman, J., St. Peter, R., and Lesser, C. 1999. Managed Care and Physicians' Provision of Charity Care. *JAMA, 281*(12), 1087–1092.

Dalaker, J., and Naifeh, M. 1998. *Poverty in the United States: 1997*. U.S. Bureau of the Census Series P60–201. Washington, DC: U.S. Government Printing Office.

Ellwood, M., and Ku, L. 1998. Welfare and Immigration Reforms: Unintended Side Effects for Medicaid. *Health Affairs, 17*(3), 137.

Fishman, L.E., and Bentley, J. 1997. The Evolution of Support for Safety-Net Hospitals. *Health Affairs, 16*(4), 30–47.

Fronstin, P. 1998. *Sources of Health Insurance and Characteristics of the Uninsured: Analysis of the March 1998 Current Population Survey*. EBRI Issue Brief No. 204. Washington, DC: Employee Benefit Research Institute.

Fronstin, P. 1999. Both Job-Based Health Coverage and Uninsured Continue to Rise. *EBRI Notes, 20*(2), 4–9.

Fronstin, P. 2000. *Sources of Health Insurance and Characteristics of the Uninsured: Analysis of the March 1999 Current Population Survey.* EBRI Issue Brief No. 217. Washington, DC: Employee Benefit Research Institute.

Gaskin, D., Hadley, J., and Freeman, V. 2001. Are Urban Safety Net Hospitals Losing Medicaid Maternity Patients? *Health Services Research,* forthcoming.

Gold, M., Sparer, M., and Chu, K. 1996. Medicaid Managed Care: Lessons from Five States. *Health Affairs, 15*(3), 153–166.

Gray, B. 1998. Hospital Ownership Form and Care of the Uninsured. *In: The Future U.S. Health Care System: Who Will Care for the Poor and Uninsured?* Altman, S., Reinhardt, U., and Shields, A. (eds.). Chicago, IL: Health Administration Press.

Health Care Financing Administration. 1999. *Medicaid Managed Care Enrollment Report, Summary Statistics as of June 30, 1998* [WWW document]. URL http://hcfa.gov/ medicaid/ trends98.htm (accessed February 14, 2000).

Hoag, S., Norton, S., and Rajan, S. 1999. *Effects of Medicaid Managed Care Demonstrations on Safety Net Providers in Hawaii, Rhode Island, Oklahoma, and Tennessee.* Princeton, NJ: Mathematica Policy Research, Inc.

Holahan, J., Rangarajan, S., and Schirmer, M. 1999. Medicaid Managed Care Payment Rates in 1998. *Health Affairs, 18*(3), 217–227.

Hurley, R., and McCue, M. 1998. *Medicaid and Commercial HMOs: An At-Risk Relationship.* Princeton, NJ: Center for Health Strategies, Inc.

Immigration and Naturalization Service. 2000a. *INS Releases Updated Estimates of U.S. Illegal Population* [WWW document]. URL: http://www.ins.usdoj.gov/graphics/publicaffairs/ newsrels/illegal.htm (accessed February 29, 2000).

Immigration and Naturalization Service. 2000b. *State Population Estimates: Legal Permanent Residents and Aliens Eligible to Apply for Naturalization* [WWW document]. URL: http:// www.ins.usdoj.gov/graphics/aboutins/statistics/lprest.htm (accessed February 29, 2000).

Internal Revenue Service. 1998. *Internal Revenue Service Announcement 98-788.* Washington, DC: Internal Revenue Service.

InterStudy. 1997. *The Interstudy Competitive Edge 7.1, Part III: Regional Market Analysis.* Bloomington, MN: InterStudy Publications.

InterStudy. 1998. *The Interstudy Competitive Edge 8.2, Part III: Regional Market Analysis.* Bloomington, MN: InterStudy Publications.

InterStudy. 1999. *The Interstudy Competitive Edge 9.1, Part III: Regional Market Analysis.* Bloomington, MN: InterStudy Publications.

The Kaiser Commission on the Future of Medicaid. 1997. *Medicaid Facts: Medicaid and Managed Care.* Washington, DC: The Henry J. Kaiser Family Foundation.

The Kaiser Commission on Medicaid and the Uninsured. 1998a. *Choices Under the New State Child Health Insurance Program: What Factors Shape Cost and Coverage?* Policy Brief. Washington, DC: Henry J. Kaiser Family Foundation.

The Kaiser Commission on Medicaid and the Uninsured. 1998b. *Market Facts.* Washington, DC: The Henry J. Kaiser Family Foundation.

The Kaiser Commission on Medicaid and the Uninsured. 1999. *Medicaid Enrollment and Spending Trends.* Washington, DC: The Henry J. Kaiser Family Foundation.

The Kaiser Family Foundation/Health Research and Educational Trust. 1999. *The 1999 Annual Employer Health Benefits Survey.* Menlo Park, CA: The Henry J. Kaiser Family Foundation and Health Research and Educational Trust.

Kalkines, Arky, Zall and Bernstein, LLP. 1999. *The Health Care Safety Net: Preserving Access to Care for Low-Income New Yorkers.* New York, NY: Kalkines, Arky, Zall and Bernstein, LLP.

Keane, C., Marx, J., and Ricci, E. 1999. Privatization and the Scope of Public Health: A National Survey of Local Health Departments. Working paper. Graduate School of Public Health, University of Pittsburgh, Pittsburgh, PA, August 19, 1999

Ku, L., and Coughlin, T. 1995. Medicaid Disproportionate Share and Other Special Financing Programs. *Health Care Financing Review, 16*(3), 27–54.

Kuttner, R. 1998. The American Health Care System: Health Insurance Coverage. *JAMA, 340*(2), 163–168.

Langreth, R. 1998. After Seeking Profits from the Poor, Some HMO's Abandon Them. *Wall Street Journal*, April 7, section B1.

Lefkowitz, B., and Todd, J. 1999. An Overview: Health Centers at the Crossroads. *Journal of Ambulatory Care Management, 22*(4), 1–12.

Legnini, M., Anthony, S., Wicks, E., Meyer, J., Rybowski, L., and Stepnick, L. 1999. *Summary of Findings: Privatization of Public Hospitals.* Washington, DC: Economic and Social Research Institute.

Lewis-Idema, D., and Bryant, S. 1998. *Trends in Medicaid and Uninsured Users Served by BPHC Grantees, 1995–1997.* Report to the Bureau of Primary Health Care, Health Resources and Services Administration. Wheaton, MD: MDS Associates.

Lipson, D., and Naierman, N. 1996. Effects of Health System Changes on Safety-Net Providers. *Health Affairs, 15*(2), 33–48.

Lipson, D., Norton, S., and Dubay, L. 1997. *Health Policy for Low-Income People in Florida.* Washington, DC: The Urban Institute.

Maloy, K.A., and Pavetti, L. 1998. *Diversion as a Work-Oriented Welfare Reform Strategy: The Experiences of Five Local Communities.* Washington, DC: Center for Health Policy Research, The George Washington University.

Maloy, K.A., Rosenbaum, S., Darnell, J. and Silver, K. 1998. *Results of a Multi-Site Study of Mandatory Medicaid Managed Care Enrollment Systems and Implications for Policy and Practice.* Washington, DC: Center for Health Policy Research, The George Washington University.

Mann, J., Melnick, G., Bamezai, A., and Zwanziger, J. 1997. A Profile of Uncompensated Hospital Care, 1983–1995. *Health Affairs 16*(4), 233–241.

Marquis, S., and Long, S. 1997. Federalism and Health System Reform. Prospects for State Action. *JAMA, 278*(6), 514–517.

MDS Associates. 1999. *The Contribution of Reconciliation Payments to Total Medicaid Revenue Received by BPHC Grantees in 1998.* Washington, DC: MDS Associates.

Medicare Payment Advisory Commission. 1999. *Report to the Congress: Medicare Payment Policy.* Washington, DC: Medicare Payment Advisory Commission.

Meyer, J., Legnini, M., Fatula, E., and Stepnick, L. 1999. *The Role of Local Governments in Financing Safety Net Hospitals: How Vulnerable to Change?* Washington, DC: Economic and Social Research Institute.

Mishel, L., Bernstein, J., and Schmitt, J. 1998. *The State of Working America, 1998–1999*, p. 243. Washington, DC: Economic Policy Institute.

Mittler, J., Gold, M., and Lyons, B. 1999. *Managed Care and Low-Income Populations: Four Years' Experience with the Oregon Health Plan.* Kaiser/Commonwealth Low-Income and Access Project. Washington, DC: The Henry J. Kaiser Family Foundation.

National Association of Community Health Centers. 1998. *1998 Survey of Community Health Centers.* Washington, DC: National Association of Community Health Centers.

National Association of Community Health Centers 1999a. *Compromise Delays Phase-Out of Health Center Payment System—Orders Congressional Report on Impact and Alternative Payment Mechanisms* [WWW document]. URL: http://www.nach.com/FSA/ Federal/ Agenda/PPS/Compromise%20 Announcement.htm (accessed February 1, 2000).

National Association of Community Health Centers. 1999b. *Health Centers and the BBA: A Mixed Review on State Efforts; A Call to Federal Action.* Washington, DC: National Association of Community Health Centers.

National Health Policy Forum. 1998. *Site Visit Report: Providing Community-Based Primary Care: Nursing Centers, CHCs, and Other Initiatives.* Washington, DC: The George Washington University.

National Health Policy Forum. 1999. *Margins as Measures: Gauging Hospitals' Financial Health:* Issue Brief Number 734. Washington, DC: The George Washington University.

Needleman, J., Chollet, D., and Lamphere, J. 1997. Hospital Conversion Trends. *Health Affairs 16*(2), 187–195.

Needleman, J., Lamphere, J., and Chollet, D. 1999. Uncompensated Care and Hospital Conversions in Florida. *Health Affairs, 18*(4), 125–133.

Norton, S., and Lipson, D. 1998. Public Policy, Market Forces, and the Viability of Safety Net Providers. Occasional Paper No. 13. Washington, DC: The Urban Institute.

O'Brien, E., Shields, A., and Pollitz, K. 1999. *The Uninsured: A Report on Health Insurance Coverage in America and Considerations for Reform.* Washington, DC: Institute for Health Care Research and Policy, Georgetown University.

Reschovsky, J., and Cunningham, P. 1988. CHIPing Away at the Problem of Uninsured Children. Washington, DC: Center for Studying Health Systems Change.

Reuter, J., and Gaskin, D. 1997. Academic Health Centers in Competitive Markets. *Health Affairs, 16*(4), 242–252.

Reuter, J., and Gaskin, D. 1998. The Role of Academic Health Centers and Teaching Hospitals in Providing Care for the Poor. In: *The Future U.S. Healthcare System: Who Will Care for the Poor and Uninsured?* Altman, S., Reinhardt, U., and Shields, A. (eds.). Chicago, IL: Health Administration Press.

Rosenbaum, S., and Darnell, J. 1997. *An Analysis of the Medicaid and Health-Related Provisions of the Personal Responsibility and Work Opportunity Reconciliation Act of 1996 (PL 104– 193).* Washington, DC: Center for Health Policy Research, The George Washington University.

Rosenbaum, S., Johnson, K., Sonosky, C., Markus, A., and DeGraw, C. 1998. The Children's Hour: The State Children's Health Insurance Program. *Health Affairs, 17*(1), 75–89.

Schneider, A. 1997. *Overview of Medicaid Managed Care Provisions in the Balanced Budget Act of 1997.* Washington, DC: The Henry J. Kaiser Family Foundation.

Schwalberg, R. 1997. *The Development of Capitation Rates Under Medicaid Managed Care Programs: A Pilot Study,* Vol. 1. *Summary and Analysis of Findings.* Washington, DC: The Henry J. Kaiser Family Foundation.

Selden, T.M., Banthin, J.S., and Cohen, J.W. 1999. Waiting in the Wings: Eligibility and Enrollment in the State Children's Health Insurance Program. *Health Affairs, 18*(2): 126–133.

Shearer, A. 1998. *Hidden From View: The Growing Burden of Health Care Costs.* Washington, DC: Consumers Union.

Shields, A. 1998. *Medicaid Managed Care and Plan Performance: The Case of Pediatric Asthma.* Ann Arbor, MI: UMI Dissertation Services.

Shields, A., Peck, M., and Sappenfield, W. 1999. Local Health Departments and the Health Care Safety Net. Working paper. Washington, DC: Institute for Health Care Research and Policy, Georgetown University.

Short, P., and Banthin, J. 1995. Caring for the Uninsured and Underinsured. *JAMA, 274*(113), 1302–1306.

Smith, V. 1999. *Enrollment Increases in State CHIP Programs: December 1998 to June 1999.* Washington, DC: The Henry J. Kaiser Family Foundation.

Smith, V., Lovell, R., Peterson, K., and O'Brien, M. 1998. The Dynamics of Current Medicaid Enrollment Changes. Washington, DC: The Henry J. Kaiser Family Foundation.

State Health Notes. 1998. In the Wake of Welfare Reform: Is the "Safety Net" Shredding, or Still Strong? *State Health Notes, 19*(279), 1,5.

Swartz, K., Marcotte, J., and McBride, T. 1993. Personal Characteristics and Spells Without Health Insurance. *Inquiry 30*(1), 64–76.

Thorpe, K., Seiber, E., and Florence, C. 1998. *The Impact of Managed Care on Hospital-Based Uncompensated Care.* New Orleans, LA: Institute for Health Services Research, Tulane University Medical Center.

United Hospital Fund. 1998. *Serving the Uninsured in a Managed Care Environment* [WWW document]. URL: http://www.uhfnyc.org/archive/cur/curv3n4.html#2 (accessed March 7, 2000).

U.S. Bureau of the Census. 1999. Population Estimates for the U.S., Regions, and States by Selected Age Groups and Sex: Annual Time series, July 1, 1990 to July 1, 1998 [WWW document]. URL http://www.census.gov/population/estimates/state/sage/sage9890.txt (accessed February 2, 2000).

U.S. General Accounting Office. 1999. *Medicaid Enrollment: Amid Declines, State Efforts to Ensure Coverage After Welfare Reform Vary.* (GAO/HEHS–99–163). Washington, DC: U.S. General Accounting Office.

Wall, S. 1998. Transformations in Public Health Systems. *Health Affairs, 17*(3), 64–80.

Wang, P. 1999. *The Changing Market, Managed Care and the Future Viability of Safety Net Providers: Graduate Medical Education.* New York, NY: Greater New York Hospital Association.

Wilensky, G. 1998. Incremental Reform: The Health Insurance Portability and Accountability Act of 1996. In *The Future U.S. Health Care System: Who Will Care for the Poor and Uninsured.* Altman, S., Reinhardt, U., and Shields, A. (eds.). Chicago, IL: Health Administration Press.

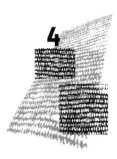

How Safety Net Providers Are Adapting to the New Environment

Safety net providers have actively been working to adjust to the new health care environment, and many have become important participants in a wide range of managed care arrangements (Kaye et al., 1999; Solloway and Darnell, 1998). As has been stated elsewhere, Medicaid programs vary widely across the states in terms of their eligibility requirements, the depth and breadth of benefits that they provide, their provider payments, and their administrative structures and processes. The diversity of their populations, the political and economic environments, their experience with managed care, and their health system infrastructure will influence the ways in which states develop Medicaid-like programs and how these programs will position safety net providers to participate and compete in the new health care marketplace (Gold, 1999; Gold et al., 1996).

A number of Medicaid managed care programs and local market conditions have proved to be particularly instrumental in shaping the direction of safety net providers' responses to the changing marketplace and potential for success (Baxter and Mechanic, 1997; Harrington et al., 1998; Norton and Lipson, 1998). The major relevant characteristics of Medicaid managed care programs of importance to safety net providers include (1) the extent of mandatory full-risk contracting, (2) the scope and speed of implementation, (3) the degree of contracting and other protections for safety net providers (e.g., procedures for enrollment and default assignment), and (4) payment policies. Key market factors of relevance to safety net providers include (1) the level of Medicaid managed care penetration, (2) the degree of competition for Medicaid patients, (3) the scope of consolidation and conversion in the local health care market and the level of for-profit health care organization, (4) the relative strengths and weaknesses of local and state policies that support of vulnerable populations, and (5) safety net providers' relative market share.

Researchers at the Alpha Center surveyed safety net providers in 10 communities, representing 6 states, to assess how these providers perceived the relative importance of market forces and Medicaid program policies on their ability to succeed in the more competitive environment (Alpha Center, 1998). Survey results showed substantial differences in how hospitals and other safety net providers view the influence of these different factors in obtaining contracts. Hospitals saw local market conditions and their own organizations' strengths and weaknesses as the key determinants of contracting success. Federally qualified health centers (FQHCs) and local health departments (LHDs) also recognized the importance of their organizations' strengths and weaknesses but viewed state and local Medicaid policies as more influential to their survival.

States have adopted managed care to control their Medicaid budgets, expand access to health care for the uninsured population, and make health care providers and health plans more accountable for performance and quality (Horvath et al., 1997; Iglehart, 1995). Individual states may prioritize these overall objectives differently (Wooldridge et al., 1997). For example:

- The state of Hawaii, with the lowest number of uninsured people in the nation, moved to mandated Medicaid managed care enrollment primarily to slow the growth of Medicaid costs and to improve the integration of Medicaid and other state programs for low-income vulnerable populations.
- Rhode Island's Section 1115 waiver program (RIte Care) was implemented to expand benefits and coverage for uninsured children and pregnant women with family incomes of 250 percent of the federal poverty level. As part of the waiver, a health plan of community health centers (CHCs) with a long track record of serving vulnerable populations was established.
- Tennessee moved rapidly to Medicaid managed care to avert a major budget crisis and to address the problem of large numbers of people without insurance.[1]

---

[1]As this report was being completed, TennCare's future fiscal viability was in significant jeopardy unless major funding to operate the current $4.3 billion program covering 1.3 million people became available. This latest crisis in the program's stormy 6-year history was generated by a December, 1999 announcement by Blue Cross Blue Shield that they would no longer participate in the program unless the state assumes some of the risk of covering TennCare enrollees. Blue Cross covers about half of TennCare's enrollees (Conover and Davies, 2000).

These different priorities can influence both how states implement their managed care programs and how safety net providers respond to new requirements and incentives.

Given the diversity of the nation's safety net, few generalities can be made about how and in what form safety providers are participating in managed care. However, the highly competitive health care marketplace is making it virtually mandatory for safety net providers to do so (Harrington et al., 1998; Lipson, 1997). With most states (the exceptions are Alaska and Wyoming) having implemented managed care programs, nonparticipation in managed care is a viable option only for safety net providers that have a unique market niche or that operate in immature managed care environments. This chapter reviews the current Medicaid managed care marketplace, some of the leading strategies safety net providers are pursuing to respond to managed care, the key elements of successful adaptation to managed care, and the major lessons being learned.

THE CHANGING MEDICAID MANAGED CARE MARKETPLACE

Although federal Medicaid regulations require states to ensure access to traditional safety net providers, managed care programs can nonetheless reduce the levels of Medicaid beneficiary utilization of safety net providers and the Medicaid revenues for these providers through a variety of means. Program design features, special waivers, or ambiguous state contractual requirements can serve to limit safety net provider participation in managed care programs (Alpha Center, 1998; Rosenbaum, 1997). Given the continuing pressure to increase states' flexibility in designing managed care programs, existing financial and guaranteed-access protections may be substantially modified or diminished.

Additional pressures for safety net providers transitioning to managed care have come from the conversion in many states from the voluntary to mandatory enrollment of Medicaid beneficiaries in managed care plans.[2] In some markets this transition has taken place very rapidly, providing less time for safety net providers to prepare and to solidify relationships with patients before the competitors of safety net providers try to enroll patients in the competitors' plans (Harrington et al., 1998). The design of state enrollment and assignment policies can also facilitate or hamper safety net providers' relationships and participation in managed care.

---

[2]In 1998, 37 states (82 percent of states with risk programs) reported mandatory rather than voluntary risk programs (Kaye et al., 1999).

An important aspect of the changing Medicaid market is the change in the trend in managed care plans' participation in Medicaid. Between 1993 and 1996 the expansion of state Medicaid managed care programs together with increasing competition for existing market share attracted the interest of many large commercial plans that had not previously participated in Medicaid (Felt-Lisk and Yang, 1997). During that period the number of commercial plans participating in Medicaid increased from 160 in 1993 to 335 in 1996, resulting in a net gain of 189 plans participating in Medicaid (some plans left the market or were acquired by other plans). Since 1996, however, a number of large commercial plans have exited this market, citing low reimbursement rates, the difficulties and high cost of administering Medicaid programs, and the complexity of Medicaid regulations (BNA's Health Care Policy Report, 1998; Hurley and McCue, 1998). A 1998 follow-up study in 15 high-volume Medicaid managed care markets by Felt-Lisk (1999a) showed a 15 percent decline in the rate of participation in Medicaid by commercial plans from 1996 to 1998.

The exit of commercial plans has been accompanied by rapid growth in the number of Medicaid-only or Medicaid-dominated plans. These diverse plans tend to be smaller; more than half of these plans have less than 25,000 members, and only 15 percent have more than 50,000 enrollees (44 percent of all full-risk managed care organizations have more than 50,000 enrollees) (Felt-Lisk, 1999b). Approximately one-half of these plans are provider based, with hospitals being the most common type of provider-owner. A growing number of these plans are owned and operated by traditional safety net providers, and these are represented by a wide variety of organizations, alliances, and approaches to managed care (Gray and Rowe, 2000). CHCs, public hospitals, other hospitals, and academic medical centers all sponsor substantial minorities of these plans.

Some policy makers have expressed concern that the decline in the level of commercial plan participation in Medicaid may jeopardize states' ability to offer "mainstream" plans to most Medicaid enrollees. Others suggest that current withdrawals may just represent a natural evolution or shakeout of the Medicaid managed care market. Despite considerable turnover in the commercial plans that participate in Medicaid, commercial plans retain a key role in serving Medicaid enrollees, even in states where multiple plans have withdrawn from Medicaid managed care (Felt-Lisk, 1999a). As the market continues to change and evolve, more research is needed on how participation in Medicaid by commercial plans influences access to mainstream care and how market instability may be affecting quality of care (Kaye et al., 1999).

SAFETY NET PROVIDER PARTICIPATION IN MANAGED CARE

The resolve by safety net providers to participate in managed care has chiefly been motivated by the growing competition for Medicaid patients and revenues. This competition has been further sharpened in the face of declining national Medicaid rolls (Holahan et al., 1998). Over the years, Medicaid became the engine that enabled CHCs to expand their services for both beneficiaries and the uninsured population. In 1980, Medicaid revenues represented only 14 percent of health center operating revenues; by 1997 that proportion had increased to 34 percent (Hawkins and Rosenbaum, 1998).

Preservation of Medicaid revenues has thus become critical to the survival of many safety net providers and, concomitantly, their ability to provide health care for the vulnerable population. By actively seeking and participating in managed care contracting, safety net providers have four major goals: (1) to maintain or expand their patient and revenue bases, (2) to reap the potential financial benefits of risk contracting, (3) to increase leverage in the Medicaid market and benefit from economies of scale through networking and other collaborative efforts, and (4) to maintain the ability to continue to serve uninsured individuals.

In striving to achieve these goals, safety net providers have identified several strategies directed to the following:

• seeking contracts with the state or managed care organizations (MCOs) on either a partial- or a full-risk basis;

• networking, affiliating, or merging with partners to gain leverage for managed care contracting and also to benefit from economies of scale that partnering can provide;

• implementing strategies and programs to diversify funding streams;

• developing and putting in place administrative and clinical protocols to improve performance and accountability;

• enhancing customer-oriented services to increase patient satisfaction and loyalty;

• making infrastructure and capital improvements designed to create attractive and efficient locations for patients to receive medical care on a regular basis;

• realigning medical staff and employees to improve productivity and to meet managed care requirements; and

• influencing the external environment by increasing advocacy efforts at all levels of government to receive more financial support.

Although it has become virtually essential for all safety net providers to pursue these strategies, the missions, roles, and competitive positions of different safety net providers make some adaptive mechanisms more important than others.

Federally Qualified Health Centers and Other Ambulatory Care Providers

In 1998, 65 percent of the nation's FQHCs participated in managed care—nearly a 16 percent increase over the previous year's level (Bureau of Primary Health Care, 1998). Most clinics contract for primary care only, thereby avoiding arrangements that would place them at risk for services not provided by the center, such as specialty services and hospital-based care (Harrington et al., 1998; Lewin-VHI, Inc., 1996).

CHCs are often viewed as important providers in managed care networks because of their geographic locations, primary care capacities, and culturally sensitive services, as well as because of the special infrastructure and expertise they have developed to serve the Medicaid population and those with special needs (Kalkines, Arky, Zall and Bernstein, LLP., 1998; Lipson and Naierman, 1996; West, 1999). The ability of CHCs to offer such important enabling services as transportation, case management, and translation also is viewed as desirable. Representatives from health centers contend that since they typically operate on constrained budgets, they have ample experience in managing the utilization of services to control the costs of care (Rosenbaum et al., 2000). Centers are now being asked to demonstrate these qualities in the new marketplace.

For many community-based safety net providers, the advent of managed care has demanded a virtual re-creation of their legal, organizational, clinical, and financial bases. Without much prior experience, providers have been asked to assume direct and legal financial risks as part of their contractual relationships with MCOs. In some parts of the United States, this dramatic conversion has taken place at a very rapid pace, with potentially dire consequences for those that do not participate or that do not meet managed care's expectations (Darnell et al., 1995).

In seeking managed care contracts, CHCs have focused their efforts on developing alliances and networks,[3] ranging from the "messenger

---

[3]As defined by the American Hospital Association, a network is a group of providers, insurers or community agencies that work together to coordinate a broad spectrum of services to their community. An alliance is a formal organization, usually owned by shareholders or members, that works on behalf of its individual members in the provision of services and products and in the promotion of activities and ventures (Moscovice et al., 1999).

model"[4] organization for negotiating managed care contracts to full-risk MCOs. By 1998, more than 50 percent of CHCs nationwide participated in some kind of managed care provider network (Harrington et al., 1998). Partnerships and networks are viewed as helping centers gain better access to self-paying patients covered by private insurance and financial resources, as well as affording them a greater chance to continue to serve existing Medicaid patients (Lipson and Naierman, 1996). By diversifying the services that they provide CHCs view the potential of attracting a broader array of patients and funding streams (e.g., funds for public employees, state corrections systems, and the State Children's Health Insurance Program). Joint ventures also help centers to invest as a group in information and quality monitoring systems, which are deemed essential tools for successful managed care contracting.

Twenty-five CHC-owned health plans are in operation in 19 states; six have the largest slice of the Medicaid market in their communities (Rhoda Abrams, Health Resources and Services Administration, personal communication, December 1999). Some of these CHC-owned plans and other aspects of CHCs and FQHCs are described in the following sections.

Community Health Plan of Washington

One of the best known CHC-owned plans is the Community Health Plan of Washington (CHPW), with approximately 50 percent of its 140,000 members enrolled in Medicaid managed care (Nichols et al., 1997). According to Dennis Braddock, the plan's chief executive officer, formation of the plan "has brought a sense of security and financial stability to the participating centers" (Dennis Braddock, CHPW, interview, November 1998). Unlike most other networks, the CHCs contract only with CHPW. According to Braddock, the plan has benefited the CHCs by assuming contractual risk, and savings are returned to the CHCs to expand and extend clinic operations and develop new facilities. The plan assumes risk for all but primary care services. CHPW contracts with non-FQHC clinics, but contracts with FQHCs for a majority of its enrollment (80 percent).

Neighborhood Health Plan

Another example of effective horizontal integration is the Neighbor-

---

[4]The messenger model is a method of setting fees for loose, non-risk bearing MCOs. A designated agent must act as a "messenger," shuttling individual physician information to the payer and vice versa. This method meets the criteria of antiturst laws that bar physicians from sharing any practice or fee information (Casualty Actuarial Society, 2000).

hood Health Plan (NHP) in Massachusetts. NHP, which became operational in 1988, is a licensed not-for-profit health maintenance organization (HMO) that serves most communities in the state. In partnership with 45 CHCs and other providers, NHP provides comprehensive health care and coverage to 107,000 members. As the largest Medicaid HMO in the state, NHP contracts with more than 140 subscriber groups representing a broad range of public- and private-sector businesses (Robert Master, Neighborhood Health Plan, Massachusetts site visit testimony, June 1998). Looking ahead at an increasingly competitive Medicaid environment, NHP became an affiliate of Harvard Pilgrim Health Care[5] in 1998 as a way of maintaining market share and adequate resources for infrastructure development. Most of NHP's participating CHCs still are being paid on a primary care case management (PCCM) or capitated primary care basis. The leadership of NHP is encouraging some of the stronger CHCs to move to full capitation, in the belief that a community-based primary care infrastructure can be more cost-effective than hospital-based ambulatory care. The issue of risk-taking was discussed during a committee site visit with executive directors of some of NHP's major participating community health centers.[6] Several of the participants expressed concerns about assuming more risk and addressed the potential advantage of affiliating with a local hospital system that can help provide the needed capital for facility and system improvements. According to Jackie Jenkins Scott, executive director of Boston's Dimock Community Health Center, "Most CHCs work on small, or no margin. Under those circumstances if you make the wrong call, you are putting your constituency at risk" (Jackie Jenkins Scott, Dimock Community Health Center, June 1998).

Rural Health Care Group

The challenge of adequately responding to today's more competitive environment with no or very limited cash reserves was underscored again during the committee's July 1998 site visit to the Rural Health Care Group, Incorporated (RHCG) in northeastern North Carolina. RHCG operates in a rural service area of 100,000 people, a quarter of whom use RHCG as

---

[5]On December 8, 1999, the state of Massachusetts agreed to purchase Harvard Pilgrim's seven medical centers for $147.6 million and then lease the centers back to the insurer. Harvard Pilgrim, which insures 1.2 million people in Massachusetts, Maine, and New Hampshire, had an estimated revenue loss of $100 million in 1999 (Jacob, 1999).

[6]Present at the June 24, 1998, meeting were representatives from Dimock Community Health Center, Great Brook Valley Community Health Center, Greater New Bedford Community Health Center, East Boston Neighborhood Health Center, and the Massachusetts League of Community Health Centers.

their primary care provider. In 1998 the center had a $10 million budget, with 76 percent of its patients receiving Medicare or Medicaid coverage; 16 percent being uninsured; and 8 percent having commercial coverage. Jane McCaleb, medical director of RHCG, pointed out that the center's major problem was a lack of financial reserves, stating, "Our daily costs are $27,000, our reserves $4,000" (amounting to approximately two hours of operation in an emergency). Inadequate reserves and the inability to purchase needed technical assistance were inhibiting the center's ability to respond to the demands of a rapidly changing marketplace. "You can't afford to spend time or dollars to move in what may turn out to be the wrong direction," was a theme echoed at other committee workshops and site visits. Although the work of the Health Resources and Services Administration (HRSA) in providing technical assistance to CHCs was considered valuable, the committee heard extensive testimony on the importance to CHCs and other safety net providers of more personalized technical assistance specifically targeted to the special circumstances of local providers and their market environments.

Primary Care Development Corporation

As another part of its fact-finding, the committee conducted a workshop in New York City, in January 1999, sponsored by The Commonwealth Fund. The committee heard a presentation on New York City's Primary Care Development Corporation (PCDC), a unique initiative that provides access to capital financing to increase the primary care capacity for medically underserved communities in New York City.[7] PCDC programs work from the principle that safety net providers must fundamentally change the way that they do business to survive in a more cost-competitive, less regulated market. Established in 1993 and supported with city, state, federal, and private-sector grants, PCDC has provided low-cost loans to 28 facilities and increased the primary care capacity so that health care can be provided for more than 700,000 patients. Each funded project also receives technical assistance. PCDC began developing technical assistance programs in 1997 and has found that "striking operational improvements are possible even among the best providers."

The underlying premises in the creation of PCDC were that primary care would be at the core of the new managed care delivery system and that primary care providers could sustain themselves through patient care revenues. An associated premise was that adequate payment rates would be developed for the effective and efficient delivery of care. All of

---

[7]Testimony of Ronda Kotelchuk, executive director, PCDC.

these premises are now being questioned by PCDC as funded projects realize smaller and even negative margins and the risk of doing business becomes ever greater. The rising number of uninsured individuals in New York City is taking an added toll on providers and the vulnerable populations that they serve. PCDC showed preliminary evidence that uninsured individuals may be receiving less primary and preventive care as community-based ambulatory care providers operate under increasing fiscal pressures.

CareOregon

In Oregon, a group of safety net providers—Oregon Health Sciences University, the Multnomah County Health Department (in Portland), and a number of CHCs—formed CareOregon in 1994 to provide care for patients in the Oregon Health Plan (OHP). CareOregon highlights some of the challenges of providing care to a disproportionate share of the high-risk patients in an environment of growing competition for Medicaid beneficiaries who are relatively healthy. CareOregon, which provides health care for 15 percent of the enrollees in the OHP, reports that it provides services to 50 percent of OHP's patients with human immuno-deficiency virus (HIV) infection or AIDS (Oregon Department of Administrative Services, 1999). Although a risk-adjusted payment methodology is beginning to be introduced, these reforms may not adequately compensate for the dramatically reduced Medicaid managed care reimbursement that the state's FQHCs now receive under Oregon's Section 1115 waiver, which no longer requires Medicaid or the plans with which it contracts to pay "reasonable" costs to FQHCs. In addition, belt-tightening measures have been introduced for OHP to compensate for the rising costs and declining cigarette tax revenues that help fund the plan. The cutbacks are reported to have had some negative spillover effects on safety net providers such as CareOregon that find themselves with a weakening ability to care for those who remain uninsured (BNA's Health Care Policy Report, 1998).

Status of Community Health Centers Under Different Participation Strategies

A Mathematica Policy Research study for HRSA looked at how FQHCs in eight national markets were faring under different participation strategies, specifically in the areas of plan and network formation (Harrington et al., 1998). Many of these efforts received start-up funds from the Bureau of Primary Health Care of the U.S. Department of Health and Human Services. Most plans and networks in the study were local in nature, reflecting historic affiliations of network providers facing the same market conditions; were not-for-profit organizations; and had at least seven members. The major findings were as follows.

- FQHCs opt to form plans to gain greater control of the funding stream and to potentially achieve greater savings, which requires them to take on greater risk. Many of the networks have a long-term goal of reducing their dependence on Medicaid enrollment and gaining Medicare and commercial contracts.

- There is an assumption that participating health centers will contribute substantial numbers of Medicaid enrollees to the network and manage costs effectively.

- In states that do not require participating plans to be licensed HMOs, networks are favoring a provider-sponsored organization (PSO)[8] instead of an HMO strategy. PSO formation tends to be less capital intensive and is viewed as offering a more gradual transition to managed care. Furthermore, PSOs allow members to focus more on their provider role and mission of serving vulnerable populations. Some states have more limited entry requirements for PSOs compared to HMOs, which tends to make the PSO model attractive to providers.

- The more successful centers appeared to be those that are larger, have a secure market niche, are led by people with strong managed care expertise, are housed in adequate facilities and have solid operating and information systems, or are supported by strong local programs for vulnerable populations.

- There are few hard rules on how centers should participate in managed care, but they cannot avoid participating at some level.

- All of the FQHCs were seeing more uninsured patients, reflecting increases in the number of both former Medicaid and now uninsured individuals and new uninsured patients. With growing numbers of uninsured individuals, FQHCs will require continued and expanded support for uncompensated care to replace some of the disappearing cross-subsidies that in the past have helped support such care.

The results of the Mathematica study suggest that FQHCs should give strong consideration to the inclusion of non-FQHC plans and pro-

---

[8]PSOs were created by the Balanced Budget Act of 1997 as a new way for providers to participate in both Medicare and Medicaid managed care programs. They are risk-bearing entities sponsored and operated primarily by providers that contract directly with Medicare and Medicaid to deliver care to beneficiaries and are often referred to as "Safety Net Plans."

viders (e.g., community-oriented commercial health plans and local hospital systems) in their MCOs as a way for centers to access capital, good information and operating systems, and support for start-up plans. The report points out, however, that such partnerships may make it more difficult for health centers to survive over the longer term as independent, community-run organizations.

Mathematica Policy Research and the Urban Institute are also involved in a 5 year research project to evaluate five Medicaid state health reform initiatives that are being conducted as Section 1115 waiver research demonstrations.[9] A February 1999 report includes information on how FQHCs in these states fared in managed care contracting between 1993 and 1996 (Hoag et al., 1999). The study found that centers across states had little or no in-house experience or knowledge base with which to negotiate managed care contracts. Contrary to FQHCs' fear that MCOs might not want to contract with them, FQHCs in all states were able to secure contracts. Nevertheless, the ability of centers to negotiate contracts was limited and many ended up with rates far below previous Medicaid rates.

The study found that safety net providers "coped" with the implementation of Medicaid managed care, but their ability to continue to evolve will be critical to their long-term survival. Using Uniform Data System data, the study found that with the exception of Oklahoma, total Medicaid revenues and Medicaid revenues per Medicaid user increased between 1993 and 1996 (Hoag et al., 1999). However, FQHCs in three of the four states had negative financial margins (as did FQHCs in the nation as a whole) in 1996 (Hoag et al., 1999). The study suggests that the FQHCs' worsening financial conditions could have been spurred by a number of factors, including additional service costs (e.g., requirements for 24-hour coverage), additional administrative costs, and the cost of caring for a greater number of uninsured patients. The study authors call for a multifaceted approach to ensuring the preservation of FQHCs, an approach that includes financial assistance, either permanent or temporary, together with technical assistance to help centers improve their business and administrative functions and develop new business arrangements (for example, partnerships with other providers).

A study for the Bureau of Primary Health Care by The Lewin Group holds similar findings. As a follow-up to an earlier study, The Lewin Group conducted a descriptive study to examine the effects of CHCs in a

---

[9]The five state projects being evaluated are Hawaii's QUEST, Rhode Island's RIte Care, Tennessee's TennCare, Oklahoma's SoonerCare, and Maryland's Health Choice.

managed care environment in seven sites across the country (Savela et al., 1998). The study concludes that the long-term survival of CHCs will rest on their ability to quickly become effective negotiators, risk evaluators, and risk managers. To achieve these objectives, centers will need to develop or procure the skills to evaluate contracts and to become effective financial managers.

The study by The Lewin Group included interviews with managers of MCOs that had contracted with the CHCs over the year to hear their perspectives on the centers' relative strengths and weaknesses within their networks. Managers lauded the expertise of their participating centers in serving the Medicaid community, their strategic importance to the individual MCO network, the centers' reputation within the community, and the centers' ability to offer more services in one location in a family practice rather than hospital-based model. Perceived weaknesses included a greater turnover of the physicians employed by the centers, a lack of sufficient extended hours compared with those for private physician groups, 24-hour coverage that is sometimes inadequate, and deficiencies in establishing timely patient eligibility and documenting services.

Other studies on how CHCs are faring and adapting show similar but uneven results, which is not surprising given the transitional environment, the changing dynamics of local markets, and the still early stage of many of these ventures at the time of study. Although managed care is being widely implemented and CHCs are able to participate in the managed care market, most centers continue to participate only on a partial-risk basis. In addition, the burden of retrenched wraparound funding (such as that received by FQHCs) has not yet affected many CHCs. Virtually every study points to the value of moving to a system with more accountability, greater performance standards, greater competition, and more choice. At the same time, evidence indicates that in the future, if current trends continue, safety net providers will need some level of special support to maintain their missions of caring for the growing numbers of uninsured individuals (Hoag et al., 1999; Kalkines, Arky, Zall and Bernstein, LLP, 1998; Lipson and Naierman, 1996; Norton and Lipson, 1998; Wooldridge et al., 1997).

Safety Net Hospitals

Public hospitals are seeking to capitalize on their strengths while also recognizing the need to lower their costs, seek broader revenue streams, and make major infrastructure investments that will help them compete for patients and revenues. Public hospitals have long been perceived to be too expensive and inefficient, and major efforts are being made to cut costs dramatically while keeping quality at an acceptable level (Bovbjerg and Marsteller, 1998). Successful adaptation to the new demands of the marketplace poses particular challenges for institutions that now need to be competitive without abandoning their mission to provide care for those who are unable to pay.

The price-driven competitive health care system has raised questions about the future of public hospitals, especially in light of excess capacity in the rest of the system. One camp views public hospitals as expensive and inefficient anachronisms that should be modified or dismantled. Another contends that, absent the public safety net functions that these hospitals perform, the most vulnerable patients in society would be left without access to health care. The truth may be somewhere in between: public hospitals will continue to be needed for their essential role but must adapt to new times (Davis, 1996; Lagnado, 1997).

Hospitals usually have a greater ability than community clinics to invest in strategic market responses (Feldman et al., 1997). In the fight for survival, many safety net hospitals are marshaling substantial planning and financial resources into restructuring and revamping their operations with an eye toward cost-cutting, downsizing, increasing productivity, and reengineering the workforce to make it more efficient and responsive to new market requirements. These priorities often involve difficult operational and personnel changes for which there has been less impetus in the past.

Changing Governing Status

The requirements of mandated managed care have moved a number of public hospitals to change their governing status to respond more flexibly and effectively. For example, in 1998 Tampa General Healthcare converted from public to private not-for-profit status to participate in joint ventures, reduce redundancies, and achieve economies of scale in purchasing, administration, and inpatient care (Bruce Siegel, Tampa General Healthcare, Florida site visit testimony, April 1998). As another example, the Boston Medical Center resulted from a merger between the publicly owned Boston City Hospital and the private, nonprofit Boston University Hospital. Cambridge Hospital—once run as an agency of the Cambridge city government—acquired Somerville Hospital and became a private nonprofit organization called the Cambridge Public Health Commission. These two new organizations remain heavily committed to vulnerable populations. Both provide approximately 50 percent of their services to Medicaid-eligible and uninsured patients; the two hospitals provide almost 60 percent of the uncompensated hospital care administered in the Boston area (Norton and Lipson, 1998).

Colorado's largest safety net provider, Denver Health, has restructured its vertically integrated system. Concerned that the constraints of the city's administrative and personnel structures were hampering Denver Health's ability to respond quickly to changes in the health care market, the hospital requested and received administrative independence from the city and became a public authority (Norton and Lipson, 1998). The Children's Hospital, the University Hospital, and the network of CHCs formed Colorado Access, the state's largest and most successful Medicaid HMO. Denver Health has a well-integrated system for efficiently addressing the needs of vulnerable populations with its network of specialty ambulatory care clinics, school-based clinics, a substance abuse detoxification facility, a local health department, an acute-care hospital with a full level one trauma center, and an HMO (Gabow, 1997).

Other safety net hospitals are placing a major emphasis on vertical integration to enhance their stake in primary care- and ambulatory care-based services. Sixty-seven percent of National Association of Public Hospitals and Health Systems member hospitals (and 69 percent of other teaching hospitals) are pursuing integration (Solloway and Darnell, 1998). To capture a share of the Medicaid managed care market, these hospitals either are forming partnerships with CHCs and other providers to develop their own HMOs or are positioning themselves to be essential providers for health plans in their regions. In Seattle, Washington, the largest provider of charity care, Harborview Medical Center, aligned with the University of Washington and the University of Washington Medical Center to create CareNet, a health plan to serve the Aid to Families with Dependent Children/Temporary Assistance to Needy Families (AFDC/TANF) population. The Washington Physician Network, comprised of Harborview and University of Washington physicians, includes a host of primary care providers (including seven clinics) and serves as the primary care base for CareNet (Norton and Lipson, 1998).

Additional Financial Assistance

Public hospitals in some of the country's major cities have received substantial financial assistance as part of their Section 1115 waivers. For example, the Los Angeles County Department of Health Services (LACDHS) received special revenues totaling $900 million over 5 years, under the condition that it reduce its inpatient capacity and reengineer its overall system to produce services at lower costs. In addition, LACDHS is using some of its waiver revenues to purchase services for its indigent populations from existing private clinics (Zuckerman et al., 1998). These federal dollars were granted in part because of an impending financial crisis in 1995 that threatened to close Los Angeles's major safety net provider. In addition to LACDHS, New York City public hospitals received approximately $100 million in additional funding for each of 5 years to prepare for the transition to managed care. In Massachusetts, Cambridge Hospital and Boston Medical Center received $70 million in federal funds to develop prepaid health plans for the uninsured.

Competitive Advantage of Safety Net Hospitals

Safety net hospitals have a number of attributes that hold potential to give them some competitive advantage in the new marketplace. Until now competition for Medicaid patients has focused on the AFDC/TANF population, with less competition for the Supplemental Security Income population and for patients with complex health care needs who are traditionally major users of safety net hospitals. Public hospitals in partnership with community-based outpatient settings have demonstrated experience in addressing the medical and social needs of vulnerable populations as they cycle on and off insurance.

Public hospitals are also focusing much attention on making their facilities more attractive and user friendly. Broader choice under Medicaid enables many beneficiaries to change plans if they are dissatisfied. Testimony heard by the committee during the California and New York City regional meetings underscored the efforts that public hospitals are making to develop attractive medical homes for their patients (Joel Cantor, New York regional meeting testimony, January 1999; David Kears, California regional meeting testimony, December 1998).

Challenges Faced by Safety Net Hospitals

Although many safety net hospitals are adapting effectively to the demands of Medicaid managed care, some systems face major barriers. Although safety net hospitals in Section 1115 waiver demonstration states (e.g., Hawaii, Rhode Island, Oklahoma, and Tennessee) participate in managed care in a variety of ways, all reported increased administrative costs as a result of increasing administrative burdens and changes in business practices imposed by either the demonstration program or market changes (Hoag et al., 1999). Financial losses were also reported by hospitals in three of the states (all but Hawaii).

Despite supplementary federal funding to help public hospitals transition to managed care, New York City's Health and Hospital Corporation projected that it would have a fiscal year 2000 deficit of $60 million (BNA's Health Care Policy Report, 1999). The deficit is being driven by the combined factors of (1) the shift from voluntary to mandatory managed care, (2) the growing numbers of uninsured—Health and Hospital Corporation cared for 495,000 uninsured people in 1999, up from 460,000 in 1998—and (3) declining reimbursement from government payers (Rick Langfelder, Health and Hospital Corporation, personal communication, March 2000).

Many safety net hospitals in Texas are facing an uphill battle in adapting to Medicaid managed care, given their inexperience in contracting with other plans, the growing competition for Medicaid patients, the stagnant if not declining local funding for care for the indigent population, and the state's general lack of supportive policies for safety net providers. A recent report on Health System, a public hospital system in urban Bexar County, Texas (San Antonio), highlights both the promise and the problems of the new funding environment (Begley et al., 1999). In response to a more competitive market for Medicaid patients, the Health System has been moderately effective at restructuring and establishing a managed care HMO that serves both Medicaid and privately insured patients, as well as a managed care product for uninsured individuals. The level of enrollment in the Medicaid HMO has been below expectations, primarily because of competing PCCM plans that appear to be more attractive to potential enrollees. Lack of primary care providers is impeding the goal of offering uninsured individuals a place to receive regular medical care; most of these patients are still seen in clinics. State-imposed marketing restrictions were found to be another important factor limiting enrollment growth (Begley et al., 1999).

TennCare has had a major financial impact on Memphis, Tennessee's, leading public teaching hospital, the Regional Medical Center, colloquially referred to as "The Med." Under TennCare, traditional safety net providers typically have not received any special consideration in managed care contracting (Gold, 1999). In efforts to expand coverage, TennCare suspended disproportionate care hospital and graduate medical education payments and reduced payments for Medicaid services. Although some of this funding was eventually restored, the temporary suspension of payment resulted in a loss of $20 million for the state's academic health centers in 1995 and a weakened ability to care for the indigent population (Meyer and Blumenthal, 1996).

The sudden and dramatic changes ("trial by fire") imposed by TennCare propelled The Med as well as the state's other academic health centers to develop strategies to deal with the challenges of reform and managed care. These strategies included the sale of clinical services through networking and product line development, reducing the costs of producing clinical services and of education and research, and improving community responsiveness and patient-customer services (Meyer and Blumenthal, 1996). Despite some positive outcomes, Medicaid revenues for academic health centers declined dramatically and increased competition has resulted in adverse selection (Gold, 1999). As an example, deliveries at The Med decreased from 8,000 to 4,000, and 3,500 of these were for high-risk pregnancies (Meyer and Blumenthal, 1996).

Safety Net Providers Operating in Rural Areas

Although Medicaid managed care enrollment is growing at an explosive rate in other parts of the country, in many rural areas HMOs are still struggling to take root. A recent survey of Medicaid officials in all 50 states suggests that to date there is little evidence that HMOs can save money in rural markets (Slifkin et al., 1998). Mandatory fully capitated programs appear to be less common in rural counties than in urban counties (10 versus 23 percent) because of provider resistance, inadequate provider supply, and other market dynamics. Rural communities are likely to have an undersupply rather than an oversupply of hospitals and physicians. Some 237 rural community hospitals closed from 1981 through 1989; during the last 3 years of that period more than two-thirds of all community closures nationwide were in rural communities (Wysong et al., 1997). Thus, although Medicaid HMOs have had their greatest impacts in cities by cutting expensive emergency department and inpatient hospital use, in rural areas without excess capacity, Medicaid patients often just forego care (Slifkin et al., 1998).

Many states, however, are determined to overcome these obstacles at least partially and have taken flexible approaches to implementing Medicaid managed care in rural areas. Programs that work in metropolitan areas cannot simply be extended to rural markets without modification. The move to managed care is also being propelled by MCOs in neighboring urban locations; in order acquire contracts with major employers, MCOs must be able to serve employees in all locations where the company operates. Such inroads by large commercial plans, however, can pose a threat to the stability of fragile local delivery systems, particularly safety net providers (Wysong et al., 1997).

Most rural states have initially concentrated on developing PCCM and partial-risk models. The expansion of primary care management programs has provided many patients with a place for regular medical care for the first time (Slifkin et al., 1998). To overcome provider resistance to managed care, states like Arkansas and South Dakota have instituted temporary case management programs that pay doctors a $2 or $3 monthly fee per patient to oversee a patient's care and that reimburse doctors on a fee-for-service basis. Other states with large rural areas (e.g., Tennessee) are easing practice restrictions and are forming strategies to supplement a meager supply of rural family physicians with the use of registered nurses and midlevel providers.

Looking at rural sites in 10 states, Mathematica Policy Research assessed the impact of managed care on rural health care providers serving low-income populations (Felt-Lisk et al., 1999). The study found that the implementation of PCCM and captitated programs is feasible even in remote rural areas but that it takes more time for the programs to accommodate to the rural health infrastructure and that they have increased difficulty in developing adequate networks. Most sites offered some protections for safety net providers, primarily in the form of cost-based reimbursement. Many providers changed their mix of services and staffing to become more efficient, maximize revenues, and better meet consumers' demands.

The Mathematica Policy Research study suggests that the move to managed care in rural areas may be improving access to primary care and creating a healthy competition for Medicaid patients. In addition, the study includes some preliminary evidence that access to specialists and hospitals may have improved for Medicaid providers, however, they have experienced increased administrative responsibilities and costs as they transitioned to managed care, and any added fees have been offset by administrative burdens. The study found that rural safety net providers in Tennessee and Oregon were having to cut back on some staff and nonmedical services and that health departments at a number of the sites were cutting back on the provision of well-child services and other clinical services. Like other studies of rural safety net providers, the impact of capitated programs on providers had no clear patterns. Safety net providers were both better and worse off depending on a combination of their market power, their proactive response, the protective payment policies available, the level of negotiated payment rates, and the specific characteristics of the state program.

Local Health Departments

The move to Medicaid managed care and competition for Medicaid patients by private providers and plans have placed many of the nation's 3,000 city and county public health agencies in a particularly vulnerable position (Martinez and Closter, 1998). As more states opt for mandatory Medicaid managed care, the revenue stream for public health departments is waning, compromising their ability to care for poor patients who do not qualify for Medicaid. In Washington, D.C., for example, where 15 publicly funded clinics once operated, only 5 remain.

For LHDs, the move to mandated managed care has brought into sharp relief the role that Medicaid program expansions have played in redirecting the core activities if not the missions of many of these agencies. Over the years, the increased availability of Medicaid funds exacerbated tensions and ambiguities that have long existed around the degree to which (if at all) LHDs should provide direct clinical services and should move away from their traditional public health functions of epidemiology and surveillance. Like other core safety net providers, LHDs have always been precariously funded, depending largely on federal, state, and local grants together with local government tax revenues. The growth in Medicaid eligibility and benefits provided incentives for many LHDs to increase their presence in direct services delivery, particularly primary care and care for special-needs populations such as individuals with HIV infection or AIDS and other infectious diseases. In many of the southern states with poor Medicaid programs or a dearth of participating providers, LHDs have long been major players in direct services delivery and are a critical component of these communities' health care safety nets (Long and Marquis, 1998). These public health agencies have proven to be well adapted to meeting the complex needs of populations that have cultural, language, educational, and other differences, such as minority and immigrant populations (Brumback and Malecki, 1996).

State Medicaid contracts generally encourage health plans to form relationships with a wide variety of public health agencies, including school-based health clinics, providers of health care for homeless people, and other providers of special services. Rarely, however, do states set specific requirements for comprehensive involvement of LHDs. Some state contracts are more likely to spell out a role for LHDs on a service-by-service basis, particularly for infectious diseases. In California, for example, the state contract specifies that patients with tuberculosis who require directly observed therapy be referred to the LHD (Zuckerman et al., 1998). For the most part, however, contracts are vague and lack clarity with respect to how health departments might be paid for services rendered, and primary responsibility for services formerly provided by health departments has shifted to managed care providers (Alpha Center, 1998; Rosenbaum et al., 1998).

As mandated Medicaid managed care continues to make inroads, public health departments are developing three distinct strategies for the creation of partnerships with MCOs, strategies that may allow them to survive and thrive in the new environment (Martinez and Closter, 1998). One strategy is to coordinate patient services and information between health departments and Medicaid managed care plans. For example, the Onondaga County Health Department (OCHD) in Syracuse, New York, established a memorandum of agreement with four LHDs for an integrated system of public health and managed care services. OCHD is reimbursed by the health plan for the population-based surveillance. Another strategy, used by Denver Health in Denver, Colorado, as well as a number of private plans, is to integrate traditional public health functions such as health promotion and disease prevention into their managed care plans.

A third strategy establishes formal systems of reimbursement for health departments and other essential community providers that are part of a managed care plan's benefits package. For example, Medicaid managed care contracts in New York City allow the LHD to provide certain screening services for which the health plan is required to pay.

Other Special Service Safety Net Providers

Other special service safety net providers (e.g., family planning clinics, school-based centers, not-for-profit visiting nurse associations, and public dental clinics) are generally experiencing much greater difficulty obtaining managed care contracts because they are not able to meet some of the key contracting provisions of managed care related to staffing and coverage. For example, under most state laws, provider groups seeking managed care contracts must prove their ability to offer a full range of primary care services and 24-hour care, a difficult hurdle for many special service providers.

A survey of community-based safety net organizations, primarily special service providers operating in Connecticut, offers some interesting perspectives (Grogan and Gusmano, 1999). Two-thirds of the safety net providers that responded to the survey said that they were participating in the state's Medicaid managed care program. The circumstances under which these organizations are participating vary widely, and this variation extends to how they are reimbursed (e.g., capitation versus fee-for-service) as well as the relative adequacy of the payment rates that they receive. The survey found that having favored legal status under the state's managed care laws does not automatically guarantee managed care contracts or adequate reimbursement. The study's most important finding points to the general lack of information that a state like Connecticut has about how safety net providers are responding to system changes and how these changes are affecting the care of Medicaid and uninsured patients.

NEW FEDERAL SAFETY NET INITIATIVE

As a way to foster further innovation and integration among safety net providers, the Clinton Administration's fiscal year 2000 budget request included a 5 year $1 billion safety net initiative to provide local community grants that would enhance collaboration and cooperation as well as innovation and greater efficiency among safety net clinics and hospitals. A major objective of the initiative is to assist communities and their safety net providers in developing integrated health care delivery systems that serve the uninsured and underinsured populations with greater efficiency and improved quality of care. The budget request included $25 million as seed funding for fiscal year 2000 and $250 million per year for each of the next 4 years to finance reforms to the health care safety net in up to 100 communities around the country. The $25 million seed money for providing health care for the uninsured and underinsured populations has been appropriated under the FY 2000 U.S. Department of Health and Human Services Appropriations Act. The new program—the Community Access Program—will be administered by HRSA (Fox, 2000).

IMPORTANCE OF STATE AND LOCAL POLICIES

Whatever strategies and adaptive mechanisms safety net providers develop, state policies and the regulatory environment will ultimately determine whether these survival strategies succeed or falter. Safety net plans, particularly on the ambulatory care side, tend to be thinly capitalized, heavily reliant on Medicaid with little ability to shift costs, and relatively small in size (less than 40,000 members). They also often lack the brand-name recognition of larger commercial plans. Although some hospitals may have deeper pockets and more resources for infrastructure improvement, their legal commitment to care for the uninsured population and the community's reliance on them for high-cost, low-margin tertiary-care services place these mission-driven institutions in a poor position to compete successfully in a highly competitive, price-driven environment. Within this framework, the environment and political-social culture in which safety net providers operate remain critical factors.

A growing number of states are fostering contracts between plans and traditional providers (Kaye et al., 1999). A 1998 survey by the National Academy of State Health Policy found that Medicaid agencies are more likely to encourage plans to contract with traditional providers than they are to require them to do so. The survey found that states are most likely to require plans to contract with FQHCs and encourage but not require contracts with other traditional providers (Kaye et al., 1999).

Most of the states studied by the Urban Institute's Assessing the New Federalism program have included special measures in the Medicaid managed care initiatives that are aimed at encouraging commercial health plans to include safety net providers in their networks or facilitating the creation of managed care plans centered on safety net providers (Coughlin et al., 1998). Minnesota requires all plans that serve Medicaid beneficiaries to include FQHCs, rural health centers, and LHDs in their networks. California, Michigan, Florida, New York, and Washington award bonus points to the bids of managed care plans when they contract with safety net providers. New Jersey and Massachusetts encouraged safety net providers to form their own plans and sought Section 1115 waivers to seek exemption from the 75/25 enrollment requirement.[10] Other states provide incentives to MCOs to contract with safety net providers by requiring that health plans meet specific access criteria (e.g., geographic primary care availability) or service criteria (e.g., family planning, targeted case management, and the provision of enabling services) that safety net providers are especially well-qualified to deliver. Some states have used automatic enrollment and automatic assignment policies to help the participation of safety net providers in managed care arrangements. For example, in California's Two-Plan model managed care initiative Medicaid beneficiaries who do not choose a plan are automatically enrolled in the "local initiative" safety net provider plans. Regardless of state incentives and requirements, many health plans recognize the unique value of contracting with safety net providers as part of their strategy to increase market share.

Given the ongoing evolution and diversity of local health care markets, it is difficult to come to any definitive conclusions regarding the priority strategies that safety net providers will need to pursue to succeed in the new environment. As part of its research, expert hearings, and meetings with key officials, the committee developed and field tested a list of characteristics and capabilities that are viewed as necessary for safety net organizations to succeed in today's challenging environment (see Box 4.1).[11] It was clear that successful adaptation goes well beyond simply participating effectively in managed care. Like any other successful health care enterprise, the successful safety net provider needs excellent leadership, financial viability, community support, patient-focused quality care, the ability to diversify its funding streams, and access to capital.

In summary, most safety net providers are developing or participating in a variety of managed care programs, including networks, affiliations, or stand-alone managed care programs, to compete effectively in the Medicaid managed care arena. Overall, these providers are experiencing some success in obtaining risk-based contracts. Many safety net providers are making concerted efforts to assume broader risk, negotiate

---

[10]The 75/25 rule, which required that 25 percent of a plan's enrollment be privately insured, was waived by the BBA of 1997 and replaced with a number of required managed care safeguards that states must build into their programs if they are to receive federal funding (see Chapter 1).

[11]The committee developed the information contained in Box 4.1 through a deliberative process using the literature, expert hearings, and regional testimony. In each case, a list of common factors was developed and field tested to establish content validity in consultation with key informants from across the nation representing safety net providers, MCOs, and state and local authorities.

BOX 4.1 Safety Net Providers: Keys to Successful Adaptation and Future Viability in a Managed Care Environment

Excellent Leadership
- Undertakes new ventures or initiatives
- Responds pro-actively to new challenges
- Recognized and respected by other key players
- Is able to participate in local and state health care decision making
- Operates effectively in a competitive, political environment
- Has attributes that reflect persistence and durability
- Operates with a board that includes business expertise

Ensures Financial Viability
- Operates with revenues exceeding expenses
- Ensures access to all funding streams
- Cost competitive for comparable services
- Manages risk

Viewed as an Important/Integral Part of the Community
- Demonstrates value-added services (viewed as among the top tier of providers in the relevant market)
- Communicates effectively with the community
- Consistent spokesperson for the uninsured population

Patient/Service Oriented
- Understands patient health care delivery preferences
- Effectively translates and implements patients' service requirements (e.g., patient hotline, language translation, extended hours, security)

Performance Oriented
- Recruits and retains quality providers and staff
- Accesses specialized services
- Attracts a diverse provider network
- Documents and performs well on recognized performance/quality and disease management standards
- Measures and improves patient satisfaction
- Holds providers and staff accountable for quality, patient satisfaction, and productivity

Develops Ability and Capacity to Be Part of a Competitive Network/ Partnership
- Has operational flexibility
- Understands components of cost
- Produces comparable cost and revenue reports

Ability to Diversify Funding Streams
- Develops other lines of business (product diversification) while maintaining the mission
- Provides important subspecialty and niche services (e.g., trauma, burn, intensive care, community and immigrant health, Children's Health Insurance Program, state employees health program, prison health)

Ability to Access Capital for Needed Infrastructure/Capacity Development
- Good physical plant/medical facilities
- Standard information and information management systems for the industry

more favorable capitation rates, aggressively preserve their Medicaid base, and establish revenue replacement strategies. The ease or difficulty in achieving these objectives appears to be closely related to the state in which these providers operate, the design of the Medicaid program, and the types of Medicaid populations covered by mandatory enrollment (Norton and Lipson, 1998). However, virtually across the board, safety net providers are seeing more uninsured patients while at the same time they are experiencing a decrease in overall levels of reimbursement, in the number of people eligible for Medicaid, and in the subsidies that have helped finance care for indigent populations. Whether in the future safety net providers can respond to the new market requirements and achieve a viable balance between margin and mission may ultimately determine whether poor people in the United States continue to receive access to health care.

REFERENCES

Alpha Center. 1998. *Medicaid Managed Care and Safety Net Providers: A Technical Assistance Guide for Managed Care Organizations*. Princeton, NJ: Center for Health Care Strategies, Inc.

Baxter, R., and Mechanic, R. E. 1997. The Status of Local Health Care Safety Nets. *Health Affairs, 16*(4), 7–23.

Begley, C., Setzer, J., Lairson, D., Masotti, P., Ribble, J., De Nino, L., and McCandless, R. 1999. *Strategies of a Public Hospital System Under Medicaid Managed Care*. Princeton, NJ: Center for Health Care Strategies, Inc.

BNA's Health Care Policy Report. 1998. Losses Driving Some Managed Care Organizations Out of Medicaid. *BNA's Health Care Policy Report, 6*(39), 1579–1582.

BNA's Health Care Policy Report. 1999. City Public Hospitals Project Deficit from Medicaid Managed Care Revenue Drop. *BNA's Health Care Policy Report, 7*(12), 516.

Bovbjerg, R., and Marsteller, J. 1998. *Health Care Market Competition in Six States: Implications for the Poor*. Paper No. 17. Washington, DC: The Urban Institute.

Brumback, C., and Malecki, J. 1996. Health Care Reform and the Role of Public Health Agencies. *Journal of Public Health Policy, 17*(2), 153–169.

Bureau of Primary Health Care. 1998. Uniform Data System. Bethesda, MD: Bureau of Primary Health Care/Health Resources and Services Administration, U.S. Department of Health and Human Services.

Casualty Actuarial Society. 2000. *Glossary of Terms in Managed Health Care* [WWW document]. URL: http://www.casact.org/health/glossary.htm (accessed March 20, 2000).

Conover, C.J., and Davies, H.H. 2000. *The Role of TennCare in Health Policy for Low-Income People in Tennessee*. Occasional Paper No. 33. Washington, DC: The Urban Institute.

Coughlin, T., Wiener, J., Marsteller, J., Stevenson, D., Wallin, S., and Lipson, D. 1998. *Health Policy for Low-Income People in Wisconsin*. Washington, DC: The Urban Institute.

Darnell, J., Rosenbaum, S., Scarpulla-Nolan, L., Zuvekas, A., and Budetti, P. 1995. *Access to Care Among Low-Income, Inner-City, Minority Populations: The Impact of Managed Care on the Urban Minority Poor and Essential Community Providers*. Washington, DC: Center for Health Policy Research, The George Washington University.

Feldman, R., Baxter, R., and Omata, R. 1997. *Staying in the Game: Health System Change Challenges Caring for the Poor*. Fairfax, VA: The Lewin Group.

Felt-Lisk, S. 1999a. *The Changing Medicaid Managed Care Market: Trends in Commercial Plans' Participation*. Washington, DC: The Henry J. Kaiser Family Foundation.

Felt-Lisk, S. 1999b. *The Changing Medicaid Managed Care Market: The Characteristics and Roles of Medicaid-Dominated Plans*. Washington, DC: Mathematica Policy Research, Inc.

Felt-Lisk, S., and Yang, S. 1997. Changes in Health Plans Serving Medicaid, 1993–1996. *Health Affairs*, 16(5), 125–133.

Felt-Lisk, S., Silberman, P., Hoag, S., and Slifkin, R. 1999. Medicaid Managed Care in Rural Areas: A Ten-State Follow-up Study. *Health Affairs*, 18(2), 238–245.

Fox, C.E. 2000. *Availability of Funds for Grants for the Community Access Program* (DOCID: fro4fe00-99) [WWW document]. URL: http://. wais.access.gpo.gov (accessed March 13, 2000).

Gabow, P. 1997. Denver Health: Initiatives for Survival. *Health Affairs*, 16(4), 24–26.

Gold, M. 1999. Insight from Oregon and Tennessee: The Influences of State Context on Medicaid Initiatives and Health Care for Low-Income Populations. Pp. 199–221. In: *Access to Health Care: Promises and Prospects for Low-Income Americans*, M. Lillie-Blanton, R.M. Martinez, B. Lyons, and D. Rowland (eds.). Washington, DC: The Henry J. Kaiser Family Foundation.

Gold, M., Sparer, M., and Chu, K. 1996. Medicaid Managed Care: Lessons from Five States. *Health Affairs*, 15(3), 153–166.

Gray, B., and Rowe, C. 2000. Safety-Net Health Plans: A Status Report. *Health Affairs*, 19(1), 185–193.

Grogan, C., and Gusmano, M. 1999. How Are Safety-Net Providers Faring Under Medicaid Managed Care? *Health Affairs*, 18(2), 233–237.

Harrington, M., Frazer, H., and Aizer, A. 1998. *Medicaid Managed Care and FQHCs: Experiences of Plans, Networks and Individual Health Centers*. Washington, DC: Mathematica Policy Research, Inc.

Hawkins, D., and Rosenbaum, S. 1998. The Challenges Facing Health Centers in a Changing Healthcare System, pp. 99–122. In: *The Future U.S. Healthcare System: Who Will Care for the Poor and Uninsured?* Altman, S., Reinhardt, U., and Shields, A. (eds.). Chicago, IL: Health Administration Press.

Hoag, S., Norton, S., and Rajan, S. 1999. *Effects of Medicaid Managed Care Demonstrations on Safety Net Providers in Hawaii, Rhode Island, Oklahoma, and Tennessee*. Princeton, NJ: Mathematica Policy Research, Inc.

Holahan, J., Zuckerman, S., Evans, A., and Rangarajan, S. 1998. Medicaid Managed Care in Thirteen States. *Health Affairs*, 17(3), 43–63.

Horvath, J., Kaye, N., Pernice, C., and Mitchell, E. 1997. *Medicaid Managed Care: Program Characteristics and State Survey Results*, Vol. 1. Washington, DC: Congressional Research Service/The Library of Congress.

Hurley, R., and McCue, M. 1998. *Medicaid and Commercial HMOs: An At-Risk Relationship*. Princeton, NJ: Center for Health Care Strategies, Inc.

Iglehart, J. K. 1995. Health Policy Report: Medicaid and Managed Care. *New England Journal of Medicine*, 332(25), 1727–1731.

Jacob, J. 1999. Massachusetts Bailing Out Health Plan. *American Medical News*, 42(48), 13–14.

Kalkines, Arky, Zall and Bernstein, LLP. 1998. *Safety Net Plans: The Role of Provider-Sponsored Health Plans in Maintaining the Safety Net in a Managed Care Era*. New York, NY: United Hospital Fund.

Kaye, N., Pernice, C., and Pelletier, H. (eds.). 1999. *Medicaid Managed Care: A Guide for States*, 4th ed. Portland, ME: National Academy for State Health Policy.

Lagnado, L. 1997. Inner-City Hospital Begs for Life Support. *The Wall Street Journal*, February 12, pp. B1–B2.

Lewin-VHI, Inc. 1996. An Evaluation of the Impact of the Social Security Act Section 1115(a) Waivers on Federally Qualified Health Centers. Fairfax, VA: Lewin-VHI, Inc.

Lipson, D. 1997. Medicaid Managed Care and Community Providers: New Partnerships. *Health Affairs, 16*(4), 91–107.

Lipson, D., and Naierman, N. 1996. Effects of Health System Changes on Safety-Net Providers. *Health Affairs, 15*(2), 33–48.

Long, S., and Marquis, S. 1998. The Effects of Florida's Medicaid Eligibility Expansion for Pregnant Women. *The American Journal of Public Health, 88*(3), 371–376.

Martinez, R.M., and Closter, E. 1998. *Public Health Departments Adapt to Medicaid Managed Care.* Issue Brief 16. Washington, DC: Center for Studying Health System Change.

Meyer, G., and Blumenthal, D. 1996. *The Initial Effects of TennCare on Academic Health Centers.* New York, NY: The Commonwealth Fund.

Moscovice, I., Wellever, A., and Stensland, J. 1999. *Rural Hospitals: Accomplishments and Present Challenges.* Minneapolis, MN: Rural Health Research Center, University of Minnesota.

Nichols, L., Ku, L., Norton, S., and Wall, S. 1997. Health Policy for Low-Income People in Washington. Washington, DC: The Urban Institute.

Norton, S., and Lipson, D. 1998. *Public Policy, Market Forces, and the Viability of Safety Net Providers.* Occasional Paper No. 13. Washington, DC: The Urban Institute.

Oregon Department of Administrative Services. 1999. Analysis of Oregon—Health Care Safety Net Services. Salem, OR: Oregon Department of Administrative Services; Office for Oregon Health Plan Policy and Research.

Rosenbaum, S. 1997. A Look Inside Medicaid Managed Care. *Health Affairs, 16*(4), 266–271.

Rosenbaum, S., Shin, P., Zakheim, M., Shaw, K., and Teitelbaum, J. 1998. Negotiating the New Health System: A Nationwide Study of Medicaid Managed Care Contracts. Special Report: Mental Illness and Addiction Disorder Treatment and Prevention. Washington, DC: Center for Health Services Research and Policy, The George Washington University.

Rosenbaum, S., Shin, P., Markus, A., and Darnell, J. 2000. *A Profile of America's Health Centers.* Washington, DC: The Henry J. Kaiser Family Foundation.

Savela, T., Chimento, L., and Stacy, N. 1998. *The Performance of C/MHCs Under Managed Care: Case Studies of Seven C/MHCs and Their Lessons Learned.* Fairfax, VA: The Lewin Group.

Slifkin, R., Hoag, S., Silberman, P., Felt-Lisk, S., and Popkin, B. 1998. Medicaid Managed Care Programs in Rural Areas: A Fifty-State Overview. *Health Affairs, 17*(6), 217–227.

Solloway, M., and Darnell, J. 1998. *The Impact of Medicaid Managed Care on Essential Community Providers.* Portland, ME: National Academy for State Health Policy.

West, D. 1999. Medicaid Managed Care: Linking Success to Safety-Net Provider Recruitment and Retention. *Journal of Ambulatory Care Management, 22*(4), 28–32.

Wooldridge, J., Ku, L., Coughlin, T., Dubay, L., Ellwood, M., Rajan, S., and Hoag, S. 1997. *Reforming State Medicaid Programs: First-Year Implementation Experiences from Three States.* Washington, DC: Mathematica Policy Research, Inc.

Wysong, J., Rosenthal, T., James, P., Bliss, M., Horwitz, M., and Danzo, A. 1997. *Introducing Medicaid Managed Care in Rural Communities.* Buffalo, NY: New York Rural Health Research Center.

Zuckerman, S., Coughlin, T., Nichols, L., Liska, D., Ormond, B., Berkowitz, A., Dunleavy, M., Korb, J., and McCall, N. 1998. *Health Policy for Low-Income People in California.* Washington, DC: The Urban Institute.

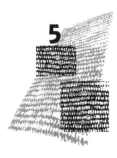

5

The Impact of Change on Vulnerable Populations

At its first organizational meeting, the committee underscored the importance of focusing its attention not only on assessing the future viability of safety net providers but also on how the major trends affecting safety net providers may affect those vulnerable populations traditionally dependent on these providers. In the committee's opinion, the future of safety net providers will depend on whether vulnerable populations will continue to believe that safety net providers can best serve their health care needs under conditions of broader choice.

As has been outlined in other chapters of this report, vulnerable populations have been shown to have broader health care needs, comprise individuals with a range of different cultural and socioeconomic backgrounds, often use a set of providers different from the providers used by the rest of the population, and have been shown to have more chronic illnesses and comorbidities. The vast majority of Medicaid beneficiaries cycle on and off insurance as their incomes and categorical eligibilities change. The new and growing phenomenon of separating care for Medicaid enrollees from care for the uninsured population may seriously compromise the potential of managed care's primary objective: to improve primary care and continuity of care. For these and other reasons the characteristics of Medicaid managed care may be fundamentally different from those of commercial managed care, given the varied and unique

aspects of individual state Medicaid programs and the special characteristics of the beneficiaries (Box 5.1).[1]

At this stage of restructuring of Medicaid managed care and health
system change, few reliable and consistent data are available to clearly
determine how vulnerable populations are faring in the new environment. Some excellent studies and surveys have been and continue to be
done in this area.[2] Almost all the study findings, however, include cau-
tions and caveats given the continuing evolution of Medicaid managed
care and the many political, economic, and policy dynamics that affect
this market. In many parts of the United States the move to Medicaid
managed care still is in an early stage, and the full impact of a more
competitive, risk-based system has not yet come into play (Holahan et al.,
1998). In addition, attempts to capture and assess the effects of current
changes on safety net clients highlight once again the wide variations
across the country in the structures and strengths of local safety net systems, the demand for their services, and the local cultures in which they
operate.

Another but related challenge is that in this turbulent market, evaluations done 3 or 4 years ago may be dated and their findings overtaken by
new policies and politics. For example, in the early 1990s, such states as
Tennessee, Oregon, and Washington planned to use the savings produced
by Medicaid managed care to increase coverage for the uninsured population (Lesser et al., 1997; Gold et al., 1995). More recently, all these states
have had to reduce such efforts in face of mounting costs or a more con-
servative political climate (Aizer et al., 1999; Marquis and Long, 1997).
The state of Rhode Island took a slower and more cautious approach
toward the implementation of its Section 1115 waiver and has been able to
further expand its coverage of previously uninsured individuals (Hoag et
al., 1999). A recent report on the evolution of TennCare illustrates a number of positive adjustments the program has made to address some of the

---

[1]The committee developed the information contained in Box 5.1 through a deliberative
process using the literature, expert hearings, and regional testimony. In each case, a list of
common factors was developed and field tested to establish content validity in consultation
with key informants from across the nation representing safety net providers, managed
care organizations, and state and local authorities.

[2]See The Urban Institute publications *Assessing the New Federalism* (Urban Institute, Washington, D.C.), which describes a multiyear project designed to analyze the devolution of
responsibility for social programs from the federal government to the states. Also see Center
for Studying Health System Change publications (Center for Studying Health System
Change, Washington, D.C.) on how the health system is evolving in 60 communities across
the United States and the effects of those changes on people. See also the Henry J. Kaiser
Family Foundation and The Commonwealth Fund series *Managed Care in Low-Income Populations: Lessons from Medicaid Managed Care in Five States.*

BOX 5.1 Characteristics of Medicaid Managed Care That Make It Different from Commercial Managed Care

Benefits
- Requires different types/levels of benefits (e.g., support services and care for a disability)
- Requires greater coordination of benefits with other financing streams
- Requires coordination with multiple levels of government and agencies to provide needed carved out (e.g., mental health and pharmacy) wraparound services (e.g., transportation and residentially based case management)
- Coverage is not continuous (i.e., on-and-off eligibility)

Population
- Special populations (e.g., populations with higher risk factors) are more prevalent and primarily comprise mothers and children
- Cultural, language, and socioeconomic differences present barriers to the provider-patient relationship; they may present logistical barriers as well (lack of a telephone, child care, and transportation)
- Individuals are less likely to have a stable source of health care
- Individuals are more vulnerable (e.g., exposed to greater levels of violence)
- Individuals have low incomes and are not in a financial position to purchase additional health care services on their own
- Individuals have a higher prevalence of behaviors that are a risk to health because of socioeconomic factors and other social inequalities
- Individuals place a lower priority on health-seeking behaviors (the emphasis is on food and housing)
- Individuals have poor self-advocacy skills

Providers
- Generally not the same provider network for Medicaid managed care as for commercial managed care; a more diverse provider network is required for Medicaid managed care
- Capitation rates for providers are often not adequate to cover the benefits or services required
- Additional burden of uncompensated safety net care for uninsured individuals
- Greater use of public teaching hospitals (e.g., for the treatment of infectious diseases and chronic conditions)
- Greater need for referrals for specialty and supportive services (e.g., substance abuse counseling and child care)
- Fewer incentives to participate as a Medicaid managed care provider because of the complexity of patient care, tenuous funding sources, and administrative requirements
- Disincentives to provide preventive services given on-and-off eligibility
- Greater administrative and oversight requirements
- Inadequate methodologies and data for accurate rate and capitation setting
- More frequent use of emergency department care, which contributes to discontinuity of care

continued

BOX 5.1 Continued

Clinical

- More chronic illness (e.g., diabetes, asthma, and high blood pressure); more comorbidities and overlays of complex social problems; more complicated pregnancies
- Greater need for mental health and substance abuse care
- Greater need for risk assessment and care management
- Inadequate quality assurance measures for complex populations
- Greater potential yield from care and case management
- Greater importance of risk adjustment
- Little or no ability to "purchase" optional or ancillary services

---

problems stemming from that state's very rapid implementation of the TennCare program in 1994 (Aizer et al., 1999). In December 1999, however, Blue Cross, which covers nearly half of TennCare's 1.3 million patients, announced that it was pulling out of the program citing inadequate funding and unstable management of the program (Page, 2000). In addition, in fiscal year 2001, TennCare is projected to have a $382 million shortfall (State Health Notes, 2000). Given the evolving Medicaid managed care market, assessments in this area appear to be particularly time-sensitive.

Despite these reservations, the existing literature provides useful insights into current trends and emerging themes as they relate to how Medicaid beneficiaries and other vulnerable populations are faring in the new health care environment. This chapter reflects on some of the leading forces driving the current environment of change and summarizes what is known to date regarding the effects of these changes on the major users of the health care safety net.

ACCESS, QUALITY, AND SATISFACTION

Access and quality of care in the traditional Medicaid program have never been optimal. The literature shows that Medicaid beneficiaries have historically faced financial and other barriers to care from private practitioners and have had to rely on emergency departments and publicly funded institutions for their health care services (The Kaiser Commission on the Future of Medicaid, 1995; The Medicaid Access Study Group, 1994). Many of managed care's principal features—its potential to strengthen preventive services and care coordination, better case management, and a clearly identifiable health care provider with overall patient management responsibilities—are generally viewed as holding promise for improving access to care for a historically underserved population. In addition, the savings that may be achieved through the use of managed care could be reinvested to improve and enhance delivery of primary care services.

Yet the very characteristics that give managed care its power also give the system a potent reason to discriminate against patients who are considered costly, difficult, or in some way "undesirable" (Rosenbaum et al., 1997). Like other managed care plans paid on a risk or capitated basis, Medicaid managed care provides financial incentives to limit beneficiary use of covered services deemed to be unneeded or inappropriate. Furthermore, because Medicaid beneficiaries may have little or no ability to choose among managed care organizations, they may be less able to express dissatisfaction by disenrolling from plans that arbitrarily deny access to needed covered services (Frederick Schneiders Research, 1996).

Incentives to economize on care could pose special problems for Medicaid beneficiaries, an economically disadvantaged group without the financial resources to purchase care directly. Many Medicaid beneficiaries reside in medically underserved areas and often have more complex health needs than higher-income Americans (Darnell et al., 1995). In addition, many Medicaid beneficiaries present with a range of other challenges, including illiteracy, inadequate social support, poor nutrition, and problems with transportation and communication, that many health plans are unprepared to address (Landon et al., 1998).

A 1995 review of the literature concluded that Medicaid managed care enrollees receive care that is at least comparable in quality to that received by their fee-for-service counterparts (The Kaiser Commission on the Future of Medicaid, 1995). More recent studies on how managed care affects access and satisfaction show mixed results. Surveys on quality and satisfaction in Medicaid managed care conducted by researchers and state Medicaid offices in a number of states (e.g., Wisconsin, Oregon, Maryland, and New York) demonstrate evidence that beneficiaries in those states are more satisfied with their health plans than fee-for-service enrollees are (CareData Reports, 1997; Oregon Department of Human Resources, 1997; Piper and Bartels, 1995; Sisk et al., 1996; United Hospital Fund, 1998). A survey of New York City Medicaid beneficiaries found that those in Medicaid managed care were more likely than their fee-for-service Medicaid counterparts to rate their medical care as excellent (13 versus 7 percent) or very good (23 versus 18 percent) (Sisk et al., 1996). A Rhode Island Department of Human Services assessment of RIte Care, presented at a May 1998 committee workshop, showed that the program had improved prenatal care and infant health outcomes (Christine Ferguson, workshop testimony, May 1998). Another study from Wisconsin indicates that the Medicaid health maintenance organizations in that state provide superior preventive care for children and have better immunization rates (Piper and Bartels, 1995).

However, findings from a Henry J. Kaiser Family Foundation survey of low-income adults in five states (Florida, Minnesota, Oregon, Tennessee, and Texas) found that Medicaid managed care enrollees were more likely than low-income, privately insured managed care enrollees to be poorer, have health problems, and experience access problems (Lillie-Blanton and Lyons, 1998). The study demonstrated that compared with the low-income, privately insured populations and Medicaid fee-for-service populations, Medicaid managed care enrollees show some improved access to a regular provider but are more likely to be dissatisfied with their health plans or experience more difficulty obtaining care.

A report on 21 focus groups that included low-income Medicaid beneficiaries in five states found that Medicaid beneficiaries' reactions to managed care depend in great part on their prior experience with seeking health care (i.e., whether they were satisfied with their previous Medicaid services) (Frederick Schneiders Research, 1996). The experiences of Medicaid beneficiaries in managed care varied widely from state to state, by economic status, by region within a state, and by other factors. Even in states where beneficiaries had positive experiences, there were problems if the switch to managed care was abrupt and poorly understood by the beneficiaries.

The most frequently cited advantage that Medicaid beneficiaries experience in managed care is improved availability of primary care, but the consistency of this trend across geographic areas and the sustainability of this trend are open to question (Felt-Lisk et al., 1997a). Improved access to primary care is closely associated with local market dynamics, rate adequacy, contractual requirements, and adequate tracking and oversight mechanisms.

Better access to primary care providers does not remove all access problems. Problems related to making an appointment, obtaining specialty care, and receiving care after hours have been cited as potential impediments to improved access. The issue of availability of care versus actual accessibility and acceptability of care needs to be clarified and better understood for the more complex and traditionally underserved Medicaid population (Billings et al., 1998; Darnell et al., 1995).

Several efforts have been initiated nationally to provide tools and performance indicators for Medicaid. These include

- the Health Care Financing Administration's Quality Assurance Reform Initiative;
- a Medicaid version of the Health Plan Employer Data and Infor-

mation Set, currently the tool most commonly used to assess health plan performance;

- the Quality Improvement System for Managed Care, designed for managed care plans that participate in Medicaid; and
- the Consumer Assessment of Health Plans (CAHP), a performance measurement instrument based on consumer reports; although the core CAHP model was designed for a general population, optional supplementary modules were also designed for Medicaid enrollees.

All of these quality assurance mechanisms are evolving, and as yet, little is known about the degree to which they will be effectively implemented or standardized across health plans or how they will affect the quality of care provided by each plan (Landon et al., 1998). John Holahan and colleagues looked at the status of Medicaid managed care quality monitoring requirements as they are being developed and implemented in the 13 states that are part of the Assessing the New Federalism project (Holahan et al., 1998). The survey found that to date there is no clear evidence of the extent to which these standards are being enforced. An early review of the impact of Section 1115 waiver programs in five states reported that none of the states had sufficient data to routinely monitor either baseline care patterns or changes in access (Gold et al., 1996).

The transitional nature of Medicaid eligibility makes quality measurement techniques more problematic. One of the major issues still to be resolved in this area is determination of the appropriate balance between federal quality assurance requirements and the flexibility of the states in designing and implementing their own programs and standards in this area.

As with other aspects of health care oversight and management, the quality oversight and management capacities of the states vary enormously. The Medicaid programs of some states are inadequately staffed to assume many of the new contracting and management functions required as Medicaid is transformed to a value-based purchaser. In implementing mandated Medicaid managed care, some states failed to recognize the importance of adequate preparation and resources for effective transition (Gold and Aizer, 2000; Gold et al., 1996). In part to compensate for uncertainties and gaps in knowledge, the federal government and states are imposing what many believe is an excessive and perhaps unproductive layer of oversight and regulatory requirements (Maura Bluestone, Bronx Health Plan, interview, December 1998; Hurley and McCue, 1998). Nevertheless, given past and more recent Medicaid marketing scandals and quality abuses, there is considerable merit in developing stringent regulations to safeguard Medicaid beneficiaries. With experience, states may be able to find a more streamlined, effective infrastructure for monitoring and oversight.

NONFINANCIAL BARRIERS TO ACCESS TO HEALTH CARE

Whereas most Americans do not require outside assistance to access and negotiate the medical system, vulnerable populations are likely to experience nonfinancial barriers that may be impediments in their search for care. These include lack of transportation and a shortage of providers in rural and inner-city areas, language and culture, and prior experiences with the medical system. Research shows that ensuring access for vulnerable populations requires consideration of both financial and nonfinancial barriers (Darnell et al., 1995; MDS Associates, Inc., 1994).

Overcoming these impediments has often been accomplished through the use of enabling services such as translation, transportation, outreach, and case management services. There is preliminary evidence that the move to capitated managed care, with its budget constraints, may affect the continued availability of outreach and other important enabling services (Felt-Lisk et al., 1997b; Hoag et al., 1999). In a more price-competitive environment, these kinds of services are more difficult to justify in the absence of hard evidence of their effectiveness and cost-effectiveness (Felt-Lisk et al., 1997b; MDS Associates, 1994). Comprehensive information on enabling services is limited, and almost no information exists on how and to what degree these services are being provided within managed care organizations (MDS Associates, 1994; R. Kotelchuck, New York regional meeting testimony, January 1999). An effort is under way to develop a mechanism for collecting and monitoring data on the utilization and costs of enabling and supportive services delivered by community-based health care providers (American Express Tax and Business Services, 1999). By developing a standardized system for the tracking of enabling services, community-based health care providers may be better able to establish their value and negotiate reimbursement for these services from payers including managed care organizations.

IMPROVING THE SCOPE AND CONTENT OF BENEFICIARY CHOICE

The issue of plan and provider choice continues to be one of the major lightning rods in the ongoing national debate over the perceived virtues and vices of managed care. The concept of choice appears to be particularly important to Americans not only in the selection of their health plan and provider but as a larger societal value. Studies and surveys on the issue of provider choice consistently indicate that people without a choice at enrollment are substantially less satisfied with their plans and managed care in general than people with choices (Fraser et al., 1998; Frederick Schneiders Research, 1996; Gawande et al., 1998). People without choice have disproportionately lower incomes and work for small employers (Fraser et al., 1998).

The Balanced Budget Act (BBA) of 1997 allows states to limit most Medicaid beneficiaries to a choice between two managed care organizations in urban areas and to a single plan in rural areas (Rosenbaum and Darnell, 1997). In neither cases does it require managed care organizations to give beneficiaries a choice among primary care physicians. Nor does the BBA of 1997 require that managed care organizations contract with physicians, hospitals, or clinics that have traditionally served low-income families and with whom Medicaid beneficiaries may have established a relationship. Nevertheless, a number of states have developed incentives for plans to include traditional safety net providers.

For the majority of Medicaid beneficiaries, who are accustomed to the fee-for-service system, learning how to navigate the managed care system and choosing a plan can be a perplexing process (Molnar et al., 1996; U.S. General Accounting Office, 1996). Investing in resources that can be used to educate beneficiaries and to counsel beneficiaries while they are choosing a plan is essential. A number of studies have looked at state education and enrollment policies and have concluded that no single consistent strategy that outlines the optimal way to inform and protect Medicaid beneficiaries as states transition to managed care can be defined (Horvath and Kaye, 1996; Mollica et al., 1996; U.S. General Accounting Office, 1996). Nevertheless, current studies and surveys help to inform beneficiaries about many of the critical issues related to education and enrollment. The key lessons that have been learned from these assessments are summarized in Box 5.2.

Many safety net providers believe that current marketing restrictions negatively affect their enrollments and detract from patients' ability to make informed choices (Kalkines, Arky, Zall and Bernstein, LLP, 1998). A study of New York City Medicaid managed care enrollees found that individuals enrolled at provider sites were far more likely than other plan members to understand plan procedures and to express satisfaction with their care (Molnar et al., 1996).

Even states with more comprehensive and sophisticated enrollment systems find that some beneficiaries are hard to reach or do not make a choice and are therefore automatically enrolled in a plan or assigned a primary care provider. Conventional wisdom has held that the voluntary versus the automatic enrollment rate is the best available indicator for measuring the effectiveness of a state's education and enrollment strategies (Maloy et al., 1998).

BOX 5.2 Lessons Learned from Managed Care Enrollment

- Although most states use the enrollment process as an opportunity to promote beneficiary understanding of the program and selection of a managed care organization, states vary significantly in their respective approaches (e.g., some states contract with outside enrollment brokers, others use dedicated staff or other state public employees, and some states make more extensive use of mailings and telephones for education and enrollment).
- Education and enrollment systems should be designed for maximum convenience and responsiveness to beneficiaries. The easier the actions required for education and enrollment, the more likely they will be used and completed. Many states have instituted mail-in enrollment, together with the availability of in-person education and counseling.
- Whether states keep their enrollment function in-house or contract with enrollment brokers appears to be less important than hiring staff whose work is dedicated to enrollment activities and services.
- In light of scandals and marketing abuses, states have turned away from letting plans do the initial marketing. More recently, states are giving enrollment brokers a more limited role and are returning some education and enrollment responsibilities back to plans, but with more oversight requirements.
- Many safety net providers believe that current marketing restrictions not only negatively affect their enrollment but also detract from their patients' ability to make informed choice given the complexity of the new managed care offerings and patients' unfamiliarity with the offerings. A study of Medicaid managed care enrollees in New York City found that individuals enrolled at provider sites were far more likely than other plan members to understand plan procedures and express satisfaction with their care (Molnar et al., 1996).
- A number of activities are necessary to acquaint beneficiaries with managed care, including outreach and follow-up capabilities. State agencies, enrollment brokers, plans, advocates, providers, and beneficiaries all have roles in outreach, marketing, and education.
- A U.S. General Accounting Office study of best practice states (i.e., Minnesota, Missouri, Ohio, and Washington) found that these states make extensive use of community-based groups and programs such as churches, Head Start programs, and maternal and child health programs in developing enrollment and disenrollment strategies.
- Variations in the time that beneficiaries are allowed to make a choice can affect their response rates.
- Rapid implementation to managed care has been associated with less knowledgeable enrollees and more chaotic transitions.
- State contracting procedures may affect continuity of care. For example, states that have a competitive bid on an annual basis and that select a limited number of plans for participation usually have more involuntary plan changes than states that engage in longer-term contracts or that allow or require all qualified plans to participate (e.g., Minnesota and Oregon).

SOURCES: Fraser et al. (1998). Horvath and Kaye (1996), Maloy et al. (1998), Mollica et al. (1996), Molnar et al. (1996), U.S. General Accounting Office (1996).

The U.S. General Accounting Office studied four states (Minnesota, Missouri, Ohio, and Washington) viewed as having effective enrollment programs (U.S. General Accounting Office, 1996). Although these "best-practice" states attempted to reach voluntary selection rates of 80 percent or higher, in their actual experiences the rates have ranged from 59 to 88 percent (U.S. General Accounting Office, 1996). Some states have automatic enrollment rates of greater than 50 percent.

Recent research indicates that understanding the dynamics of automatic enrollment and their implications for Medicaid beneficiaries is much more complex than was originally perceived. There appears to be little knowledge about whether, from a beneficiary's standpoint, automatic enrollment is associated with less satisfaction, lower rates of access and utilization, and less understanding of the managed care system (Maloy et al., 1998). Ongoing research in this area is beginning to show that automatic enrollment rates may ultimately be less important than what Medicaid beneficiaries actually experience once they enroll in a plan. For example, automatic enrollment may be less meaningful if a beneficiary's provider participates in both plans being offered or beneficiaries know that they can easily move out of a plan if they are not satisfied.

State enrollment policies often play two critical and potentially conflicting roles in Medicaid managed care, and both roles have major implications for beneficiaries. First, enrollment policies can play a vital role in the goals of educating beneficiaries about their managed care options and the selection of a plan of their choice. A high rate of voluntary enrollment is viewed by states as an indicator that the goals are being achieved. Second, automatic enrollment has been used by states as a vehicle to create a market for new start-up plans or for special classes of providers deemed important to the program. For example, such states as New York and California use automatic enrollment as a way to steer patients to safety net providers. As the Medicaid managed care market matures and states improve their enrollment practices, the rate of automatic enrollment will likely decline. In light of the recent exit of commercial plans from the Medicaid market, some states may continue to rely on automatic enrollment as a lever to attract certain plans to the program.

HOW EFFECTIVE ARE CURRENT ENROLLMENT AND CHOICE POLICIES?

The ultimate test of any education and enrollment strategy is how well it works in helping beneficiaries make informed and meaningful choices. Unfortunately, there has been a dearth of evaluations, and strong performance measures of effective education and enrollment efforts are not available (U.S. General Accounting Office, 1996). Voluntary disenrollment rates tend to be low (3 percent or less) and too small for meaningful aggregate analysis (information about individual disenrollment decisions may be more useful) (Horvath and Kaye, 1996). Until now, most state Medicaid programs have focused primarily on threshold dimensions of managed care (e.g., how managed care differs from the fee-for-service system, the difference between mandatory and voluntary enrollment, enrollment guidelines, and the scope of beneficiary protections). Although this information is useful and relevant for beneficiaries, numerous studies have shown that Medicaid patients care less about what plan they can join than about whether they will have access to a specific provider or group of providers (Ku and Hoag, 1998). However, timely and accurate participating provider lists are not routinely available to enrollees. A recent United Hospital Fund survey of New York City Medicaid beneficiaries showed that 46 percent of managed care enrollees reported that they had not received a provider list (Cantor et al., 1997). Beneficiaries are also interested in information on their covered benefits, but about 25 percent of those surveyed thought that their benefits would expire if they did not sign up for a plan (Cantor et al., 1997). A study on state enrollment systems being conducted by the Center for Health Services Research and Policy at The George Washington University found that a lack of information about providers and plan networks consistently precluded meaningful Medicaid beneficiary choice during enrollment (Maloy et al., 1998).

Medicaid beneficiaries report that their most valued and trusted sources of information about their choice of plans were their providers or community-based organizations (Maloy et al., 1998; U.S. General Accounting Office, 1996). However, although the Medicaid and uninsured populations often have an array of special needs, most states do not provide much comparative information about providers' capacities to meet those needs (Fraser et al., 1998).

MAINSTREAMING

Mainstreaming is often cited as a goal in extending managed care to vulnerable populations. The Medicaid program originally sought to bring low-income Americans into the mainstream of medical care, moving them away from their almost exclusive reliance on safety net providers. In reality, Medicaid has fallen far short of that goal. Because of its low payment rates and socially unpopular clientele, the program has for the most part failed to attract the participation of a broad range of providers, particularly for primary care (The Medicaid Access Study Group, 1994). A more price-competitive health care landscape has made Medicaid a more attractive payer to the commercial sector. To compensate for shrinking revenues, commercial plans and providers have focused on enlarging market share and the number of covered lives.

Many HMOs were initially attracted to the Medicaid market as an opportunity to quickly increase revenues, but other reasons also prevailed. Several states, including Minnesota, require HMOs to serve the Medicaid population as a condition for offering a commercial product to state employees. Plans also use the Medicaid market to expand and leverage their provider networks or as a beachhead from which they can increase their market share of other payers. Finally, certain plans participate in Medicaid to be viewed as good corporate citizens in their communities (Hurley and McCue, 1998).

In the early 1990s commercial plans had yet other incentives for commercial plans to participate in Medicaid managed care. Before 1994, enrollment in managed care had mainly remained voluntary and reimbursement rates were relatively generous (Bovbjerg and Marsteller, 1998; Hurley and McCue, 1998). Some states actively sought commercial plans' involvement in the Medicaid market as a way to mainstream low-income beneficiaries and to move away from a perceived two-tier health care system.

In a number of states the entry of commercial plans may have contributed to the broadening of access to primary care. According to focus groups, some Medicaid beneficiaries "felt the advantage of high-quality doctors" or appreciated the chance to "see mainstream providers in mainstream delivery settings" (Frederick Schneiders Research, 1996). These observations are tempered by evidence and testimony heard by the committee that some beneficiaries return to seek care from their traditional providers with whom they feel more comfortable and accepted (Kalkines, Arky, Zall and Bernstein, 1998; West, 1999; Florida site visit testimony, April 1998). There appear to be no reliable data, however, on the number of Medicaid patients who leave their traditional providers to join other managed care organizations or on the number who return to traditional providers after having been enrolled in a commercial plan.

Experience is beginning to show that mainstreaming is not easily accomplished and, to the degree that it exists, that it must occur on two levels: both the plan and the provider levels (Hurley and McCue, 1998). Medicaid beneficiaries' enrollment in a commercial plan is no guarantee that they will have access to the same network of providers as their counterparts whose premiums are paid by private payers, particularly for referral and specialty care services (Marsteller, 1998). Even when states have attempted to regulate equity of access, enforcement of such provisions has proved problematic for state officials, given the technical complexity of assessing even the basic adequacy of a network (Fagan and Riley, 1998). More research is needed on how participation by commercial plans influences access to mainstream care and how it affects quality (Kaye et al., 1999).

Regardless of the intrinsic merits of mainstreaming Medicaid beneficiaries as a policy objective, efforts to move in this direction may be losing some momentum. In the past 2 years, several large commercial plans have exited from all or major segments of the Medicaid market, citing rate inadequacy, rate volatility, and administrative burdens associated with government requirements, as indicated in two studies (Hurley and McCue, 1998; McCue et al., 1999). Those studies examined the financial performances of health plans and interviewed a number of Medicaid managed care plan executives. Many of the managed care plan executives admitted that their predominantly commercial plans probably would not be able to surpass the growing Medicaid-only plans in customizing their services for Medicaid beneficiaries. These executives expressed concern, however, over the long-term ability of Medicaid-only plans to provide high-quality care for their beneficiaries given these providers' dependence on Medicaid revenues and their having to accept whatever rates would be meted out.

Traditional safety net providers have claimed that they see more patients with greater health risks than do their counterparts in commercial plans. There is some evidence that when marketing to Medicaid beneficiaries commercial plans focus their efforts on the healthier segments of this population, particularly pregnant women (Gaskin et al., 1998). A recent study examining the services and status of Oregon's health care safety net conducted by Milliman and Roberston for the Office for Oregon Health Plan Policy and Research sheds some additional light on this question (Oregon Department of Administrative Services, 1999). The study's findings confirm that, in general, both safety net and mainstream clinics find Medicaid patients to be more difficult to serve. The study found, however, that the state's safety net plan, CareOregon, and its clinics saw a sicker population than mainstream plans in three categories and that the reimbursements that these providers received were low relative to the costs of providing such care. In addition, although enabling services were offered in both mainstream plans and CareOregon, the study suggests that safety net clinics are more effective than mainstream clinics at delivering enabling services to Medicaid patients who have special needs.

Another study comparing the quality management practices of health plans participating in Medicaid managed care found that Medicaid plans are more likely than commercial plans to target programs directed to the specific needs of the Medicaid population (Landon and Epstein, 1999). The study concludes, however, that neither commercial nor Medicaid plans showed notable strong records in actual quality improvement.

The results of the analysis of the Oregon health care safety net as well as other research highlight the importance of adequate risk adjustment methodologies not only to promote fairer competition among health plans but also to help ensure that consumers have an adequate choice of providers in their markets (Bovbjerg and Marsteller, 1998). Currently, premiums are usually adjusted for age, gender, and geographic regions, but there is growing interest in adjusting payments for the health status of enrollees. More refined risk adjustment will better compensate plans that enroll higher-risk or sicker patient populations and reduce incentives for selecting only healthier enrollees. At this time only two states, Colorado and Maryland, incorporate health-based risk-adjustment systems into their capitation rates (Holahan et al., 1999). In the absence of adequate risk adjustment, states have opted to carve out certain services from health plans' benefits packages or to include stop-loss provisions in their contracts with managed care organizations.

THE UNINSURED POPULATION

By any measure, the growing number of uninsured people, 18.4 percent of the country's total nonelderly population and more than 30 percent of the nation's low-income individuals in 1998, is the most serious and troublesome by-product of the new health care paradigm. In a market-driven environment the uninsured, who do not represent a market force, are excluded.

A range of research has shown that relative to insured people, uninsured people are much more likely to have unmet health care needs, are less likely to have a usual source of care, have lower rates of health care use, and experience worse health outcomes, including increased rates of mortality. Individuals without health care coverage have long been a public policy concern for a nation whose coverage system is largely built on employment status or eligibility for publicly financed programs. The combination of eroding employment-based coverage, changing demographics, welfare reform, the shrinking ability on the part of health care providers to cross-subsidize the costs of health care, and the move to Medicaid managed care has raised the problem of this nation's uninsured to what many perceive to be a critical juncture. State programs directed at improving access for the uninsured have been developed in such states as Oregon, Washington, and Minnesota. Although these efforts have been shown to improve the levels of access, each of these programs is facing funding problems and has had to limit some of the original objectives (Lipson and Naierman, 1996).

Although most of the published literature indicates that safety net providers have been able to maintain their commitment to the uninsured population, recent anecdotal evidence indicates that a weakened safety net is beginning to reduce the standby protection for those who remain uninsured. Safety net providers are treating a growing number of uninsured patients whereas the number of paying patients is declining and the payments for them are being reduced. In some communities, uninsured patients are having to wait longer or must be sicker to get an appointment, and some services offered previously are no longer available (Baxter and Feldman, 1999). In their review of safety net hospitals and community health centers in 12 communities, Baxter and Feldman found evidence that some of these providers were being forced to limit access to health care services because of the growing demand for services for the uninsured population. Reductions in Medicaid disproportionate share hospital payments, restructuring of state charity pools in Newark, New Jersey, and Boston, Massachusetts, and the changing insurance status of immigrant populations in Miami, Florida; Orange County, California; and Phoenix, Arizona, are forcing providers in these communities to reduce the level of access for the uninsured population (Baxter and Feldman, 1999).

INNOVATIVE NEW APPROACHES TO CARE
FOR THE UNINSURED POPULATION

A positive sign on the current horizon is experimentation with managed care approaches to providing care for the indigent uninsured population. The first and best-known model for using managed care to provide access to health care to the uninsured population was established in Tampa, Florida, in 1991 (Lipson et al., 1997; Norton and Lipson, 1998). Faced with a rising number of poor workers and high-risk individuals without insurance, Hillsborough county petitioned the Florida Legislature for authority to levy a half-cent sales tax to help finance access within a coordinated system of care. Contracting on a competitive basis with networks of community health centers, hospitals, and other providers, Hillsborough HealthCare now serves an estimated 25,000 people. According to testimony heard during the committee's site visit, Hillsborough HealthCare has contributed to a marked lowering of hospitalizations for diabetes and asthma complications through improved access to primary care and reduced emergency department expenditures (Patricia Bean, Hillsborough County Health Plan, Florida regional meeting testimony, April 1998; Commissioner Thomas Scott, Hillsborough County Board of Commissioners, Florida regional meeting testimony, April 1998). For its success, the program has received the "Models that Work" award from the Health Resources and Services Administration for innovative health improvement programs. Similar programs that link uninsured people to a primary care provider or medical home to coordinate their care have been started by public hospitals in Indianapolis, Boston, and Bextar County, Texas.

The success of Hillsborough as a model that could be replicated in other parts of the country was an important catalyst behind the launching of a major new $16.8 million initiative, Communities in Charge: Financing and Delivering Health Care to the Uninsured, sponsored by the Robert Wood Johnson Foundation. The program is designed to help a broad-based consortia of organizations in the community develop and implement managed care delivery systems for low-income, uninsured individuals, emphasizing prevention and early intervention.

Similarly, the W.K. Kellogg Foundation's Community Voices program is another major philanthropic-sponsored effort targeted to sustaining, improving, and expanding health care for the uninsured populations. Begun in 1998, Community Voices seeks to ensure the survival of safety net providers and strengthen community support services, "given the unlikely prospect of achieving universal health coverage in the next 5 years" (Community Voices, 2000). Thirteen diverse communities—selected to serve some of the hardest-to-reach underserved populations—have received grants to serve as laboratories of change to sort out what works from what does not in meeting the needs of those who receive inadequate or no health care.

OTHER CHALLENGES

As previous studies have shown, although health insurance coverage is an important component of ensuring access to care, it is not the only factor. A new study that looked at changes in access to care from 1977 to 1996 indicates that during this time access to a usual source of care has declined sharply for Hispanics and young adults aged 18 to 24 (Zuvekas and Weinick, 1999). However, no more than 20 percent of the change in access could be explained by declines in rates of health insurance coverage. Demographic changes, large decreases in rates of access among the uninsured population, and, for young adults, decreased rates of access among those with insurance were shown to be important contributing factors.

Other dynamics associated with a more competitive, price-based environment, such as conversion, consolidation, and privatization, in the future may add new pressures to an already tenuous national capacity to serve the vulnerable and uninsured populations. Although recent reports on conversions and privatization indicate that access for low-income patients is not yet seriously degraded, those studies and surveys attest to a changing and unstable environment that requires more active attention and monitoring (Needleman et al., 1997).

As part of the new managed care requirements and as a means of survival in a more competitive environment, traditional providers are being compelled to place greater emphasis on performance, development of a more customer-responsive environment, and more efficient operations. To the degree that improvements in this area continue, the move to managed care will benefit the care of the nation's most vulnerable citizens. Inadequate capitation rates and declining subsidies, however, may quickly erode this potential, particularly given the rising number of uninsured people and the tenuous hold that these providers have in balancing their missions and margins.

Medicaid managed care in many ways can be likened to a halfway technology: a concept that has significant potential but one that is as yet hamstrung by programs and policies that blight the promise. Instead of pursuing mainstreaming as an objective per se, giving beneficiaries access to quality providers under conditions of informed choice may be a more relevant and meaningful goal for certain vulnerable populations. In a competitive, cost-driven marketplace and in the absence of a national policy on the uninsured population, a quality provider for vulnerable populations must be a provider or plan that will ensure some continuity of care as individuals cycle on-and-off coverage.

Only a stronger national commitment directed to the problem of the nation's growing number of uninsured people will help fulfill the true promise of managed care for America's low-income populations. Nevertheless, there will always be some Americans whose vulnerabilities and special needs will exceed the capabilities of the services that can be purchased with a health insurance card alone.

REFERENCES

Aizer, A., Gold, M., and Schoen, C. 1999. *Managed Care and Low-Income Populations: Four Years' Experience with Tenncare*. Washington, DC: The Henry J. Kaiser Family Foundation.

American Express Tax and Business Services. 1999. *Enabling and Supportive Services: Definition and Cost Calculation*. New York, NY: American Express Tax and Business Services, Inc.

Baxter, R., and Feldman, R. 1999. *Staying in the Game: Health System Change Challenges Care for the Poor*. Fairfax, VA: Center for Studying Health System Change.

Billings, J., Greene, J., and Mijanovich, T. 1998. *Analysis of Primary Care Practitioner Capacity for Medicaid Managed Care in New York City*. New York, NY: Wagner School of Public Health, New York University.

Bovbjerg, R., and Marsteller, J. A. 1998. *Health Care Market Competition in Six States: Implications for the Poor*. Paper No. 17. Washington, DC: The Urban Institute.

Cantor, J., Weiss, E., Haslanger, K., Madala, J., Heisler, T., Kaplan, S., and Billings, J. 1997. *Ambulatory Care Providers and the Transition to Medicaid Managed Care in New York City*. New York, NY: United Hospital Fund and New York University.

CareData Reports. 1997. *Medicaid HMO Survey Report*. White Plains, NY: CareData Reports.

Community Voices. 2000. About Community Voices [WWW document].URL: http://www.community voices.org/aboutcommunity.html (accessed February 28, 2000).

Darnell, J., Rosenbaum, S., Scarpulla-Nolan, L., Zuvekas, A., and Budetti, P. 1995. *Access to Care Among Low-Income, Inner-City, Minority Populations: The Impact of Managed Care on the Urban Minority Poor and Essential Community Providers.* Washington, DC: Center for Health Policy Research, The George Washington University.

Fagan, A., and Riley, T. 1998. *The KAISER-HCFA State Symposia Series: Transitioning to Medicaid Managed Care.* Portland: ME: National Academy for State Health Policy.

Felt-Lisk, S., Harrington, M., and Aizer, A. 1997a. *Medicaid Managed Care: Does It Increase Primary Care Services in Underserved Areas.* Washington, DC: Mathematica Policy Research, Inc.

Felt-Lisk, S., Harrington, M., and Aizer, A. 1997b. *Availability of Primary Care Services under Medicaid Managed Care: How 14 Health Plans Provide Access and the Experience of 23 Safety Net Providers and their Communities.* Washington, DC: Mathematica Policy Research, Inc.

Fraser, I., Chait, E., and Brach, C. 1998. Promoting Choice: Lessons from Managed Medicaid. *Health Affairs,* 17(5), 165–174.

Frederick Schneiders Research. 1996. *Medicaid and Managed Care: Focus Group Studies of Low-Income Medicaid Beneficiaries in Five States.* Washington, DC: The Henry J. Kaiser Family Foundation.

Gaskin, D., Hadley, J., and Freeman, V. 1998. *Are Urban Safety Net Hospitals Losing the Competition for Low Risk Medicaid Patients?* Washington, DC: Institute for Health Care Research and Policy, Georgetown University.

Gawande, A., Blendon, R., Brodie, M., Benson, J., Levitt, L., and Hugick, L. 1998. Does Dissatisfaction with Health Plans Stem from Having No Choices? *Health Affairs,* 17(5), 184–194.

Gold, M., and Aizer, A. 2000. Growing an Industry: How Managed Is TennCare's Managed Care? *Health Affairs,* 19(1), 86–101.

Gold, M., Frazer, H., and Schoen, C. 1995. *Managed Care and Low-Income Populations: A Case Study of Managed Care in Tennessee.* Washington, DC: The Henry J. Kaiser Family Foundation and The Commonwealth Fund.

Gold, M., Sparer, M., and Chu, K. 1996. Medicaid Managed Care: Lessons from Five States. *Health Affairs,* 15(3), 153–166.

Hoag, S., Norton, S., and Rajan, S. 1999. *Effects of Medicaid Managed Care Demonstrations on Safety Net Providers in Hawaii, Rhode Island, Oklahoma, and Tennessee.* Princeton, NJ: Mathematica Policy Research, Inc.

Holahan, J., Zuckerman, S., Evans, A., and Rangarajan, S. 1998. Medicaid Managed Care in Thirteen States. *Health Affairs,* 17(3), 43–63.

Holahan, J., Rangarajan, S., and Schirmer, M. 1999. Medicaid Managed Care Payment Rates in 1998. *Health Affairs,* 18(3), 217–227.

Horvath, J., and Kaye, N. 1996. *Enrollment and Disenrollment in Medicaid Managed Care Program Management.* Portland, ME: National Academy for State Health Policy.

Hurley, R., and McCue, M. 1998. *Medicaid and Commercial HMOs: An At-Risk Relationship.* Princeton, NJ: Center for Health Care Strategies, Inc.

The Kaiser Commission on the Future of Medicaid. 1995. *Medicaid and Managed Care: Lessons from the Literature.* Washington, DC: The Henry J. Kaiser Family Foundation.

Kalkines, Arky, Zall and Bernstein, LLP. 1998. *Safety Net Plans: The Role of Provider-Sponsored Health Plans in Maintaining the Safety Net in a Managed Care Era.* New York, NY: United Hospital Fund.

Kaye, N., Pernice, C., and Pelletier, H. (eds.). 1999. *Medicaid Managed Care: A Guide for States,* 4th ed. Portland, ME: National Academy for State Health Policy.

Ku, L., and Hoag, S. 1998. Medicaid Managed Care and the Marketplace. *Inquiry, 35,* 332–345.

Landon, B., and Epstein, A. 1999. Quality Management Practices in Medicaid Managed Care: A National Survey of Medicaid and Commercial Health Plans Participating in the Medicaid Program. *JAMA, 282*(18), 1769–1775.

Landon, B., Tobias, C., and Epstein, A. 1998. Quality Management by State Medicaid Agencies Converting to Managed Care. *JAMA, 279*(3), 211–216.

Lesser, C., Duke, K., and Luft, H. 1997. *Care for the Uninsured and Underserved in the Age of Managed Care.* New York, NY: The Commonwealth Fund.

Lillie-Blanton, M., and Lyons, B. 1998. Managed Care and Low-Income Populations: Recent State Experiences. *Health Affairs, 17*(3), 238–247.

Lipson, D., and Naierman, N. 1996. Effects of Health System Changes on Safety-Net Providers. *Health Affairs, 15*(2), 33–48.

Lipson, D., Norton, S., and Dubay, L. 1997. *Health Policy for Low-Income People in Florida.* Washington, DC: The Urban Institute.

Maloy, K., Silver, K., Darnell, J., Rosenbaum, S., Kreling, B., and Kenney, K. 1998. *Results of a Multi-Site Study of Mandatory Medicaid Managed Care Enrollment Systems and Implications for Policy and Practice.* Washington, DC: Center for Health Policy Research, The George Washington University.

Marquis, S., and Long, S. 1997. Federalism and Health System Reform. Prospects for State Action. *JAMA, 278*(6), 514–517.

Marsteller, J. 1998. *Impact of Restriction of Insurance Premiums on Rates of Insurance and Uninsurance.* Washington, DC: The Urban Institute.

MDS Associates. 1994. *Enabling Services: What We Know and What Remains to Be Learned.* Washington, DC: Office of the Assistant Secretary for Health, U.S. Department of Health and Human Services.

McCue, M., Hurley, R., Draper, D., and Jurgensen, M. 1999. Reversal of Fortune: Commercial HMOs in the Medicaid Market. *Health Affairs, 18*(1), 223–230.

The Medicaid Access Study Group. 1994. Access of Medicaid Recipients to Outpatient Care. *New England Journal of Medicine, 330*(20), 1426–1430.

Mollica, R., Riley, T., Horvath, J., and Kaye, N. 1996. *Transitioning to Medicaid Managed Care. Consumer Protection: Lessons Learned from States.* Portland, ME: National Academy for State Health Policy.

Molnar, C., Soffel, D., and Brandes, W. 1996. *Knowledge Gap: What Medicaid Beneficiaries Understand and What They Don't About Managed Care.* New York, NY: Community Service Society of New York.

Needleman, J., Chollet, D., and Lamphere, J. 1997. Hospital Conversion Trends. *Health Affairs, 16*(2), 187–195.

Norton, S., and Lipson, D. 1998. *Public Policy, Market Forces, and the Viability of Safety Net Providers.* Occasional Paper No. 13. Washington, DC: The Urban Institute.

Oregon Department of Administrative Services. 1999. *Analysis of Oregon Health Care Safety Net Services.* Salem, OR: Office for Oregon Health Plan Policy and Research, Oregon Department of Administrative Services.

Oregon Department of Human Resources. 1997. *Progress Report: The Oregon Health Plan Medicaid Reform Demonstration, Part I.* Salem, OR: Office of Medical Assistance Programs, Oregon Department of Human Resources.

Page, L. 2000. Blues Plan Throws in Towel, Leaves Troubled TennCare. *American Medical News, 43*(1), 1, 34.

Piper, K., and Bartels, P. 1995. Results from Wisconsin Suggest that HMOs Are More Effective than Fee-for-Service in Primary and Preventative Health Care. *Public Welfare, 53*(2), 18–21.

Rosenbaum, S., and Darnell, J. 1997. *A Comparison of the Medicaid Provisions in the Balanced Budget Act of 1997 (P.L. 105–33) with Prior Law.* Washington, DC: The Henry J. Kaiser Family Foundation.

Rosenbaum, S., Serrano, R., Magar, M., and Stern, G. 1997. Civil Rights in a Changing Health Care System. *Health Affairs, 16*(1), 90–105.

Sisk, J., Gorman, S., Glied, S., DuMouchel, W., and Hynes, M. 1996. Evaluation of Medicaid Managed Care: Satisfaction, Access, and Use. *JAMA, 276*(1), 50–55.

State Health Notes. 2000. TennCare: Once Again, on the Brink of Change. *State Health Notes, 21*(317), 8.

United Hospital Fund. 1998. *Utilization, Access, and Satisfaction Under Voluntary Enrollment* [WWW document]. URL: http://www.uhfnyc.org/archive/cur/ curv3n4.html#2 (accessed March 7, 2000).

U.S. General Accounting Office. 1996. *Medicaid: States' Efforts to Educate and Enroll Beneficiaries in Managed Care.* Gaithersburg, MD: U.S. General Accounting Office.

West, D. 1999. Medicaid Managed Care: Linking Success to Safety-Net Provider Recruitment and Retention. *Journal of Ambulatory Care Management, 22*(4), 28–32.

Zuvekas, S., and Weinick, R. 1999. Changes in Access to Care, 1977–1996: The Role of Health Insurance. *Health Services Research, 34*(1), 271–279.

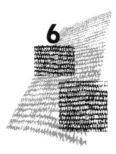

6

Safety Net Populations with Special Health and Access Needs

This chapter reviews how changes in Medicaid policy, the growth in enrollment in managed care, and the changes in the marketplace are affecting those Americans with serious chronic illnesses or disabilities as well as those who have experienced social dislocation (e.g., homeless people). These populations (hereafter referred to as special-needs populations) have special health care and access needs and are often viewed as particularly medically and economically vulnerable. The committee wanted to take a closer look at this group because it provides a unique opportunity to understand how the changing health care environment might affect the safety net and the people it serves. Policies that negatively affect those individuals with special needs are likely to have adverse effects on many other patients. Similarly, policies that serve the needs of people with special health needs are likely to positively affect other patients. The failures and successes of Medicaid policy changes, managed care, and the health care marketplace are likely to be more quickly apparent for those with special needs, such as people with serious mental illness or human immunodeficiency virus (HIV) infection/acquired immune deficiency syndrome (AIDS). Thus, the special-needs populations may provide early insights that can be generalized to all populations in the safety net system. Special-needs populations also receive attention in this report because they account for a disproportionate share of medical expenditures and they bring into greater focus a number of the challenges in the further expansion of Medicaid managed care. A closer look at this important subset of the safety net population helps illuminate issues related to contracting, financing mechanisms, adequate information systems, integration and coordination of care, and the need to bundle health care and enabling services.

This chapter examines two categories of special-needs populations: (1) nonelderly adults and children with chronic illnesses and disabilities who qualify for Supplemental Security Income (SSI) or who meet a state's medically needy standard for Medicaid and (2) adults and children who experience extraordinary access barriers because of social dislocation (e.g., homelessness, immigrant status, or language or cultural differences) and who require specially designed outreach programs to facilitate access to and utilization of basic health care services.

The committee examined four special-needs populations to highlight some of the issues related to the changes in the health care marketplace: children with special needs, people with serious mental illnesses (SMIs), people living with HIV infection or AIDS, and homeless people. These groups illustrate some of the major challenges that the chronically ill and disabled populations in the safety net system bring to the policy debate. Similarly, the homeless illustrate problems of social dislocation, that is, difficult-to-reach populations, who traditionally are cared for by safety net providers.

This chapter also brings into bold relief the fact that people with special needs are often served by specialty providers in the safety net, providers who are not well linked to the primary care providers in the system. Special-needs populations in the safety net require complex health care services and enabling or social services. Funding for the care of people with special needs is fragmented and is dependent on the annual appropriations process, contributing to a service system that has traditionally been plagued with problems of coordination and a lack of continuity between primary care and specialty care services. To successfully care for these populations, policies must ensure access to necessary and appropriate specialty medical and enabling services for this population while also bridging the gap between the primary and specialty safety net systems.

PEOPLE WITH SPECIAL NEEDS

People with Chronic Illnesses and Disabilities

Approximately 14.5 percent of the U.S. population has a disability covered by the Americans with Disabilities Act (ADA), including 6.1 percent of children under the age of 18 (Wenger et al., 1997). Any number of conditions may cause a person to be disabled, but disability is less about disease or diagnosis and more about functional capacity. Functional limitations include those things that negatively influence participation in work, school, leisure, family, and community life. People with disabilities use a wide spectrum of health and enabling services including primary care, acute care, rehabilitation, mental health, addiction, respite care, and long-term-care services. The service requirements are as diverse as the individuals who need them and may vary among those with the same conditions. There are no simple formulas for predicting service utilization, but clearly, care for the disabled population is more costly than care for the general population.

People with disabilities are broadly defined as those with limitations in human actions or life activities due to physical or mental impairments (Americans with Disabilities Act [ADA; P.L. 101–336]) (LaPlante, 1991). There is no single, up-to-date source of disability rates by diagnosis or special population, nor is there a single, comprehensive, up-to-date compilation of expenditures by diagnosis group.

People with disabilities are much more likely than their nondisabled counterparts to have publicly funded health care coverage. Half of all medical expenditures for people with disabilities are covered by public programs, including 30 percent by Medicare, 10 percent by Medicaid, and 10 percent by other public programs. This compares to a rate of publicly funded health care of only 20 percent for the nondisabled population. In addition, although it is likely that people with disabilities have some type of public insurance, many others are nevertheless uninsured. Almost 10 percent of children who need help with activities of daily living are uninsured, as are 12 to 13 percent of disabled adults (LaPlante et al., 1993; Trupin et al., 1995).

The pace of movement of people with disabilities into managed care has been dramatically slower than that of low-income women and children. Although the Balanced Budget Act of 1997 allowed states to mandate enrollment of most Medicaid beneficiaries in qualified managed care plans, children with special needs and individuals with dual eligibility (adults who qualify for both Medicaid and Medicare) were exempted. To enroll such individuals in managed care plans, states still must seek a federal Medicaid waiver from the Health Care Financing Administration. Most states did not rush to put their disabled populations into managed care plans, hoping first to learn lessons in implementing managed care for women and children before enrolling higher-risk beneficiaries. Nonetheless, all but 15 states now enroll at least some of their disabled beneficiaries in managed care plans (Figure 6.1), and several are considering doing so in the near future (Regenstein and Schroer, 1998).

In addition, all but four states have developed behavioral managed care programs that cover some combination of primary and specialty mental health services (Substance Abuse and Mental Health Services Administration Managed Care Tracking System, 1998). Early indicators

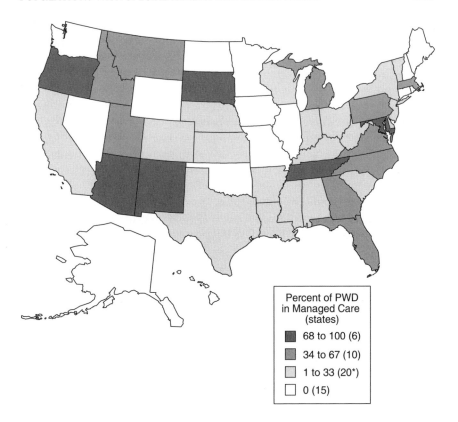

FIGURE 6.1 Percentage of nonelderly persons with disabilities (PWD) in Medicaid managed care, 1998. *Includes District of Columbia. SOURCE: Regenstein and Schroer (1998). Reprinted with permission of the Henry J. Kaiser Family Foundation of Menlo Park, California. The Kaiser Family Foundation is an independent health care philanthropy and is not associated with Kaiser Permanente or Kaiser Industries.

suggest that it is feasible to move disabled populations into managed care with some degree of success, although the risk of failure is high because of the potential interruption of essential services to a highly vulnerable population and the potential of the unraveling of the safety net for the special-needs population.

Safety net providers for this population are especially skilled in blending financial resources from multiple funding sources (federal, state, and local) to support the provision of services for the special-needs population, but Medicaid continues to be the bedrock of health care and related services for this group and provides the infrastructure of services for the special-needs population. Because disabled special-needs populations make up only 16 percent of the total Medicaid population but account for 37 percent of Medicaid (Regenstein and Schroer, 1998), states are moving in the direction of managed care for this group (Figure 6.2). Several factors have contributed to states' interest in managed care for this population:

• In comparison with Medicaid beneficiaries who also receive Aid to Families with Dependent Children, who are now covered under Temporary Assistance to Needy Families, average spending per beneficiary is higher for those with disabilities ($1,304 versus $8,168) (Bishop and Skwara, 1997).

• Medicaid spending for persons with disabilities grew at an annual average rate of 14 percent from 1990 to 1994, with growth slowing from a high of 19 percent in 1990–1991 to 9.5 percent in 1993–1994 (Bishop and Skwara, 1997).

• States vary widely in conditions of eligibility and coverage and cost per beneficiary. For example, in 1996 the annual cost per SSI beneficiary ranged from $2,846 in Tennessee to $13,320 in Connecticut (Bishop and Skwara, 1997).

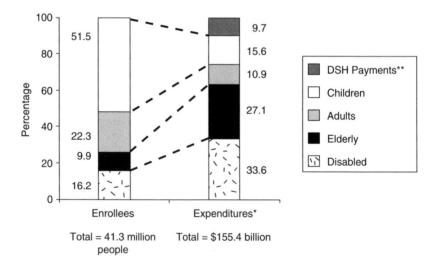

FIGURE 6.2 Medicaid enrollees and expenditures by enrollment group, 1996. *Total expenditures exclude administrative expenses. **DSH, disproportionate share hospital payments. SOURCE: The Kaiser Commission on Medicaid and the Uninsured (1999). Reprinted with permission of The Kaiser Commission on Medicaid and the Uninsured.

Liska (1997) concludes that the goal of reduced expenditures in Medicaid cannot be reached without enrolling special-needs groups in managed care since they account for such a large proportion of total program expenditures.

Whereas managed care has largely been piloted by the commercial insurance industry, important legal, structural, operational, and historic differences between Medicaid managed care and commercial managed care are highlighted by the care provided for disabled populations. Traditional insurance plans and managed care organizations do not typically provide coverage for the essential nonmedical enabling services (e.g., social and vocational rehabilitation services, transportation, and case management) that special-needs populations require and that are often provided by safety net providers. Such services, although required under Medicaid, might not be provided by Medicaid managed care plans unless the provision of such services is explicitly spelled out in the contract and is monitored through specific quality-improvement standards (Rosenbaum et al., 1998).

Somers and Brodsky (1997) noted that there are few tested models of the provision of Medicaid managed care to populations with complex health care needs because of uncertainty on the part of purchasers and plans about how to design benefits and delivery systems and coordinate with related funding streams and services for them. Their study also found inadequate rate-setting and risk-adjustment capacities and warned that a devolution of purchasing, administration, and oversight responsibilities to county governments could result in inconsistent purchasing practices and policies.

Safety net providers for special-needs populations are at potentially greater risk in a Medicaid managed care environment for several reasons. Although some of these providers can offer a comprehensive array of medical and enabling services, more often a provider of care for a special-needs population has developed a niche in highly specialized medical or enabling services funded through a combination of Medicaid and special programs such as state block grants for mental health and substance abuse services or Title V Maternal and Child Health Bureau (MCHB) block grants for children with special needs. These providers may thus be unable to provide the full range of services required to participate as a primary care provider. The packaging and financing of their services will depend on rate-setting and risk-adjustment policies that consider the special medical and enabling needs of their populations.

Children with Special Needs

Children with special needs present challenges for managed care plans with regard to rate setting and projections of service utilization because of problems with defining, and thus counting, the population. Moreover, since they represent a group more integrated into the core safety net than other special-needs groups, their primary and specialty services illustrate the potential for integrated managed care models of primary and specialty care services.

Safety net providers for special-needs children include community health centers, public hospitals, children's hospitals, school-based health clinics, public health departments, and a number of private not-for-profit specialty service agencies. Safety net funding sources include Medicaid, Title V MCHB grants combined with matching funds from the states, the State Child Health Insurance Program, Individuals with Disabilities Education Act funds, and Head Start funds (Institute of Medicine, 1996).

The two principal sources of funding for special-needs children in the safety net are Medicaid and Title V MCHB grants. Special-needs children are more likely to be covered by Medicaid than by private insurance because of the Early and Periodic Screening, Diagnosis, and Treatment (EPSDT) program included in the benefits package. The EPSDT program provides broader coverage for expanded services (e.g., for nonmedical services or access to other health professionals like nurse practitioners or nutritionists). Nationally, the average annual cost of EPSDT program benefits for healthy children is about $1,000 to $1,500, whereas it is $5,000 to $6,000 for special-needs children (Institute of Medicine, 1998). The average cost of caring for special-needs children varies greatly by state, region, and market, as does the average cost per diagnosis or service need (Alliance for Health Reform, 1997).

Title V MCHB funds are used to provide services not covered by Medicaid programs for both disabled and nondisabled children, including programs offered by local health departments and community and migrant health centers and for HIV infection prevention and treatment. Title V MCHB funds are also typically used to strengthen linkages among variously funded programs to support community-based care for children. This is especially important for special-needs children, whose care would otherwise be fragmented (Institute of Medicine, 1998).

Because children with special needs have the same need for regular developmentally appropriate primary care and immunization visits as nondisabled children, they will more likely receive care from a pediatrician, family practitioner, or some other primary caregiver (Neff and Anderson, 1995). In fact, pediatric primary care providers have been encouraged to play active roles in caring for children with chronic health conditions by acting as the coordinator of medical and related services, providing referrals to specialists when necessary, and helping families manage on a day-to-day basis (Blancquaert et al., 1992; Ireys et al., 1996; Liptak and Revell, 1989; Young and Schork, 1994). The integration of primary and specialty care is prompted by the ongoing need for regular primary care services as well as the special developmental needs of children (Kuhlthau et al., 1998). However, in some parts of the country, pediatric subspecialties are located in regional medical centers, making integration more difficult (Institute of Medicine, 1996; Schlesinger and Mechanic, 1993).

The fact that special-needs children suffer from more than 200 conditions, all with a relatively low prevalence, poses special challenges in defining the population and setting appropriate parameters for the delivery and financing of care through managed care arrangements. The problems of definition are so vexing that the MCHB Division of Services for Children with Special Health Needs established a national consensus panel, which concluded that this population is best defined by its service needs rather than by diagnosis or disability per se (McPherson et al., 1998). Medical expenditures for special-needs children account for 70 to 80 percent of all medical expenditures for children, and expenses for special needs children are, on average, five to six times higher than those for healthy children (Institute of Medicine, 1998; Neff and Anderson, 1995; Newacheck and Taylor, 1992).

By 1998, 38 states had mandated managed care arrangements for at least some children with special needs (Kaye et al., 1999). Early implementation data from programs in California and Massachusetts provide useful insights (National Governors' Association, 1996).

Like most other states, California has exempted special-needs children from the state's mandatory Medicaid managed care programs to allow time to demonstrate the feasibility and cost-effectiveness of incorporating them into the program. Pilot projects that explore different provider reimbursement models include full-risk, partial-risk, and fee-for-service case management with a variety of payment mechanisms:

- capitation payments to primary care providers, under which providers are capitated for the full scope of services or are capitated for a specific range of services;
- capitation to all providers; and
- staff model health maintenance organizations with a variety of physician payment mechanisms.

Alameda County, California, is testing a "special-needs risk factor scale" to identify Medicaid-eligible children who require additional services. The scale ranks a child in three areas: family risks, presence of medical problems, and involvement with multiple community agencies. The model seems to differentiate practices with large volumes of special-needs children from practices with small volumes. The former receive increased capitation payments (National Governors' Association, 1996).

Massachusetts enrolls children with special needs in the state's Medicaid managed care program, MassHealth. Through a grant from MCHB the state has established the Managed Care Enhancement Project, a cooperative effort between the state's Title V staff and Medicaid programs to improve the health status of special-needs children. The level of reimbursement is intended to be commensurate with the increased level of effort required to serve special-needs children (National Governors' Association, 1996).

A "special care coordinator" is assigned either to one large physician practice or to two or more smaller practices to assist with additional case management functions related to the care of special-needs children. The grant also helped fund the development of a manual for the families of special-needs children (National Governors' Association, 1996).

People with Serious Mental Illnesses

People with SMIs represent a group that is treated in a publicly financed safety net system that runs parallel to the general health care safety net. Only 20 percent of people with a mental health problem seek care through a primary care provider, and these tend to be people with relatively minor or treatable disorders (Institute of Medicine, 1997). Those with more serious mental health problems are cared for in the specialty mental health system and highlight the need for coordination of services as well as the difficulties associated with a fragmented service system.

The most serious and disabling mental disorders (schizophrenia, major depression, and bipolar illness or manic-depressive disorder) affect about 2 percent of the population annually (Institute of Medicine, 1997). Schizophrenia affects more than 2 million Americans over the course of their lifetimes and accounts for approximately 49 percent of all psychiatric hospitalizations.

Overall, the public sector bears about two-thirds of the costs of providing care for people with mental health problems, in particular, for those with the most serious disorders. The costs of treating mental illness exceed the costs of treating many other diseases and are comparable to the costs of treating cancer and cardiovascular disease (Institute of Medicine, 1997). Roughly 25 percent (about 2.6 million) of the population that qualifies for SSI is eligible because of a serious mental disorder other than mental retardation (Alliance for Health Reform, 1998). Payments from Medicaid account for an estimated 14 percent of all national spending on mental illness and addiction services, whereas payments for these services account for roughly 9.6 to 12.6 percent of Medicaid spending.

Those with SMIs represent high-need, moderate-cost users for whom recent advances in pharmacological treatment have been made, for whom a number of community-based rehabilitation interventions have been refined and the efficacies of which have been established, and who have an established need for an extensive network of enabling and case-management services to maintain or improve community-based functioning.

In general, the public mental health system has encouraged the coordination of medical and enabling services to integrate people with SMIs into the community. However, the single greatest flaw of the mental health safety net is its nearly total disconnection from the core safety net addressed in this study. Managed care holds the potential to achieve better coordination between the two systems, if not integration of the two systems.

A wide array of safety net providers serve those with SMI, including community mental health centers, state and county psychiatric hospitals, family and social service agencies, transitional living and social programs, housing and vocational rehabilitation programs, and a number of consumer-driven self-help programs. The public mental health system, like the public general health system, has a patchwork of funding streams: federal, state, and local sources including Medicaid, Medicare, federal block grants to the states, and a myriad of state and local funds targeted to various community-based not-for-profit programs. For example, community mental health centers serve clients of all income levels regardless of ability to pay, but the majority of these individuals are uninsured or are receiving coverage through some public benefit program. More than 70 percent of community mental health center revenues are from public sources, including 16 percent from Medicaid (Butler, 1993). A distinguishing feature of the public mental health safety net is that it serves as the early default system for people whose private insurance benefits run out in the course of a serious mental illness, a frequent occurrence (Institute of Medicine, 1997).

The service system largely comprises publicly funded agencies whose primary missions are delivery of psychiatric services and coordination of enabling and other services. This system is supplemented by a community-based network of private not-for-profit agencies that provide many of the special enabling services that people with SMIs require: child care, transportation, domestic violence counseling and shelter for those affected by domestic violence, housing, employment and skills training, and education. The mental health community has come to embrace these services as being equal in importance to more traditional medical services such as medication and therapy (Institute of Medicine, 1997). These services are not routinely provided by traditional managed care plans and must be carefully delineated in behavioral health managed care contracts.

A recent tracking study prepared for the Substance Abuse and Mental Health Services Administration Managed Care Tracking System (1998) by The Lewin Group reports that as of July 1998, 46 states (the exceptions are Maine, Mississippi, Nevada, and Wyoming) have implemented some type of behavioral health managed care, up from 27 states in 1996. The study indicates that safety net providers have retained a significant role in the care of people with SMIs in managed care plans. Specialty long-term care for people with SMIs is generally provided in stand-alone, carve-out, or partial carve-out plans.[1] More than half the programs are managed by public-sector agencies or private-public partnerships. More than one-third of the mental health programs cover residential, crisis, rehabilitation, and support services. Medicaid acts as the lead agency for more than half the programs, and more than half the programs target SSI beneficiaries who qualify by virtue of their mental illness. However, the study also suggests that in states that opt to integrate services (27 states), safety net providers may have a decreased presence. Furthermore, integrated managed care organizations often use a secondary carve-out contract with a behavioral health managed care organization or safety net provider to shift the financial risk. Whether or not safety net providers participate in risk contracts, this approach may increase the downward pressure on rates, threatening their future viability.

A study from the George Washington University (Rosenbaum et al., 1998) of Medicaid managed care contracts for behavioral health care found that contracts show enormous variations in the definition of terms like *outpatient care, urgent care,* or *emergency care,* leaving much room for differences in actual scope of coverage among organizations with seemingly similar contracts. In general, state agencies give contractors broad latitude in terms of coverage determination and prior authorization procedures. Many general and managed behavioral care agreements permit disenrollment of persons who are disruptive; some states specify that this

---

[1]*Stand-alone* programs refer to managed behavioral health programs independent of any other program (i.e., they are not carved out of a physical health program). *Carve-out* models completely separate behavioral health services or populations from physical health managed care programs. *Partial carve-out* models use a combined integrated approach for some behavioral health services but place other expanded services or populations under a separate managed care program. The intent is to provide a basic set of behavioral health benefits under a comprehensive physical health plan but to supplement them under a separate program for special populations whose needs go beyond those covered by the basic plan (Substance Abuse and Mental Health Services Administration Managed Care Tracking System, 1998, p. I-20).

practice is prohibited for patients whose disruptive behavior is related to the illness, like SMI.

Mechanic (1998) notes that integrated plans appear to be effective for the general population but that carve-out plans have emerged as the favored approach to the treatment of people with an SMI. He advises that if carve-out plans are inevitable, mechanisms to improve communication and better define responsibilities at the boundaries of specialty and primary care need to be developed, need to be built on interdisciplinary team efforts, and need to use well-established practice guidelines. Rosenbaum et al. (1998) found that carve-out plans create multiple tiers of coverage, responsibility, and accountability, leaving room for gaps in service to highly vulnerable populations like those with an SMI. Most notable was the recommendation to slow the implementation of managed care for disabled populations:

> The headlong rush into managed care is neither wise nor necessary. No population should be pressed into a managed care arrangement that is not ready to enroll the population carefully or provide them with care of adequate quality. The problem with rushing too quickly into managed care is especially great when the lower-income population targeted for such enrollment suffers from physical or mental disabilities and is being enrolled into companies and plans with little or no experience in the care of low-income persons with high health care needs (Rosenbaum et al., 1998, p. 73).

A recent case analysis of Tennessee's failed behavioral health managed care program underscores the caution to move slowly (Chang et al., 1998). The analysis found that Tennessee moved too quickly to implement TennCare Partners (a statewide behavioral health care carve-out plan). Among the many outcomes of the failed TennCare Partners plan was an increase in the number of people with SMIs in the state correctional system, a documented loss of about 15 percent of necessary services for people with SMIs in 1 year, involuntary medication changes as the result of problems with the plan's formulary, and high rates of disenrollment of low-cost clients, leaving the behavioral health managed care organizations with the same number of high-cost clients but substantially fewer numbers of enrollees and less revenue with which to provide care. The investigators acknowledged the potential economic and medical advantages of carve-out plans for this population but made four recommendations for states considering such carve-out arrangements:

- Behavioral health care managed systems must increase accountability and reduce the level of bureaucracy.
- Both consumers and providers should be protected with risk-adjusted

capitation payments. Enrollees must be assessed promptly, and their clinical status must be updated routinely for proper risk-adjustment purposes.

• Patients should be protected with an effective quality assurance program. This means not only that the desired outcomes and measures must be specified but also that the state must take the time to put information and data systems in place and develop mechanisms for oversight, including the capacity for periodic site visits.

• States considering the implementation of behavioral health managed care programs are encouraged to do it on a pilot basis that focuses on only a segment of the population. This avoids the risk of a major failure that is difficult to repair and allows the state to gradually learn what is appropriate to the populations being placed at risk (Chang et al., 1998, pp. 868–869).

People with HIV Infection or AIDS

HIV infection and AIDS highlight the importance of payment methodology and the problems of translating aggregate cost data to reasonable per person payments. People with HIV infection or AIDS represent a group that requires many health care services, is at risk of many health problems, and whose care is high cost, but at the individual level there is enormous variation in health care needs and costs both on an annual basis and on a lifetime basis. It is a group for which treatment standards are so rapidly evolving that it is difficult to predict the level of utilization of services and costs. As treatment and life expectancy improve for people with AIDS and the benefits of new drug therapies become known, there will be increased attention on people with HIV infection and early intervention, with implications for managed care plans. Currently, there is such wide variation in Medicaid reimbursement rates among the states that the best predictor of care for this group is the state in which they live.

In fiscal year 1999 the combined federal and state Medicaid expenditures on HIV infection and AIDS were expected to be $3.9 billion, and the Medicare expenditure was expected to be $1.5 billion (Foster et al., 1999). Medicare will play an increasing role in the support of care for people with HIV infection and AIDS as more people with AIDS survive the 29-month waiting period for Medicare coverage under the Social Security Disability Insurance (SSDI) program.[2] It is projected that Medicare pay-

---

[2]SSDI is a program administered by the Social Security Administration to provide cash assistance to certain people who have paid into the Social Security Trust Fund and who are unable to work because of a disability. Five months after the onset of their disability, disabled people can begin to collect SSDI cash benefits. After an additional 24-month waiting period (for a total of 29 months), they become eligible for Medicare coverage.

ments for HIV infection and AIDS will accelerate to $2.1 billion by the year 2002 (Fasciano et al., 1998; Pine, 1998). In addition, the Ryan White CARE Act supports a number of ongoing clinical, demonstration, and education projects for people with HIV infection and AIDS. In 1999 an estimated $1.4 billion was expended through the Ryan White CARE Act for a variety of services and demonstration projects (Foster et al., 1999).

Between 1996 and 1997 four protease inhibitors were approved by the U.S. Food and Drug Administration, adding to the growing armamentarium of drugs approved for the treatment of HIV infection and AIDS, launching a new era in the treatments for these conditions and dramatically altering life expectancies for many people with AIDS. Although before 1996 the death rate from AIDS had increased every year, in 1996 the death rate from AIDS dropped by 23 percent, and it fell by another 44 percent in the first half of 1997. The number of new cases of HIV infection has not fallen but has held steady at about 40,000 to 80,000 per year (Centers for Disease Control and Prevention, 1997; Hellinger, 1998). Improvements in early detection, increases in life expectancy, and recommended multiple-drug treatment regimens early in the course of HIV disease will create new financial burdens for patients as well as the safety net. For example, the increase in new cases and earlier treatment have placed enormous strains on already stretched AIDS drug assistance programs, which provide access to needed drug therapy for people who lack insurance coverage for such treatments, regardless of their eligibility for Medicaid or Medicare (Buchanan and Smith, 1998). It is estimated that combination drug therapy that includes protease inhibitors costs about $12,000 per person per year, and the laboratory fees associated with monitoring a patient's response to drug therapy cost another $1,400 to $1,500 per patient per year (Bartlett and Moore, 1996; Hirschel and Francioli, 1998; Moore and Bartlett, 1996).

People with HIV infection or AIDS are disproportionately male, black, and poor; 46 percent have annual incomes of less than $10,000; 68 percent have public health insurance or no insurance; and 30 percent receive care at a teaching hospital. In 1996 hospital costs were still the most expensive component of care, but the costs of pharmaceuticals were already double the amount spent on all other components of outpatient care for HIV infection and AIDS combined. Hospital expenditures are expected to continue to decline with increases in the number of available pharmaceuticals and greater use of outpatient care (Bozzette et al., 1998).

Although the total cost of care for people with HIV infection or AIDS constitutes only 1 percent of overall health expenditures, the annual per-person cost is unpredictable and can be quite high. Since Medicaid pays for more than 50 percent of direct medical care provided to adults living with HIV infection or AIDS and about 90 percent of the care provided to infected children, states are interested in managed care to provide quality care to a high-risk population and contain costs (The Kaiser Commission on the Future of Medicaid, 1996). By June 1996, 35 states reported enrolling people with HIV infection or AIDS in Medicaid managed care programs (Rawlings-Sekunda and Kaye, 1998). Several recent reports provide in-depth case studies of states that have approached managed care for this population in very different ways, depending on the concentration of people with HIV infection or AIDS in the area, geography, the availability of HIV and AIDS specialists, and the availability of cost information (Bartlett, 1998; Rawlings-Sekunda and Kaye, 1998; Health Resources and Services Administration, 1997). Two states illustrate the different challenges facing rural areas (Tennessee) with low concentrations both of people with HIV infection or AIDS and of specialists in this area of care and urban areas (Maryland) with high concentrations of both.

Tennessee's AIDS Centers of Excellence model, which is part of its TennCare program that serves all Medicaid beneficiaries, builds on the experiences of a few physicians with expertise in HIV infection and AIDS. Centers are established on the basis of expertise and experience in the treatment of HIV infection and AIDS and are fee-for-service subcontractors for all plans on a voluntary basis. There is broad participation of stakeholders in the establishment and implementation of the authority of the Centers, with special attention paid to linking medical and enabling services. Prior authorization procedures are waived for prescriptions and other treatments, and patients can elect to have the Centers act as their primary care providers (Rawlings-Sekunda and Kaye, 1998).

TennCare uses risk pools to protect plans against adverse risk selection. Each quarter the state calculates the difference between the total cost of paying for enrollees with specific conditions on the basis of Medicaid fee-for-service payments and the total amount paid to each plan for providing services to those enrollees. Each plan is reimbursed the difference unless the total costs exceed the budget, in which case the money is divided in proportion to each plan's share of the costs (Rawlings-Sekunda and Kaye, 1998).

Although the Centers of Excellence model shows promise for rural and underserved areas, its consensus building and voluntary infrastructure could disintegrate in the face of uncontrolled or escalating costs associated with the treatment of HIV infection and AIDS, a risk which will be closely monitored by stakeholders.

In July 1997, Maryland initiated a Medicaid Section 1115 waiver with mandatory enrollment of all Medicaid beneficiaries with HIV infection or AIDS. The state uses a risk-adjusted Ambulatory Care Group (ACG) reimbursement mechanism with a special capitation mechanism for people with AIDS but no special rate for those in earlier stages of HIV infection. The ACG mechanism assigns rates to non-AIDS patients, including those with HIV infection, on the basis of their recent levels of health care utilization. The rates for people with disabilities range from $95 to $1,102 per member per month. New enrollees for whom there is no utilization history are assigned rates based on gender, age, and place of residence (Health Resources and Services Administration, 1997).

Johns Hopkins University's experience with the ACG rates for HIV-infected patients was that the average cost of care for these patients is $1,000 per patient per month, whereas the average reimbursement rate was only $500 per patient per month (Bartlett, 1998; Johns Hopkins University, 1997). Care for HIV infection is delivered through a mixed model, with expertise in HIV infection and AIDS care available in mainstream plans and centers of excellence in which enrollees may see HIV and AIDS specialists for both primary and specialty care (Health Resources and Services Administration, 1997). Special capitation rates are applied to patients who meet the Centers for Disease Control and Prevention's 1993 definition of AIDS and are based on historic fee-for-service costs trended forward. The costs of protease inhibitors, specialty mental health care, viral load testing, and newly approved HIV-related drugs are carved out and paid on a fee-for-service basis. In 1998, rates were set at $2,161 for people living in Baltimore and $1,812 for people living elsewhere in Maryland (Health Resources and Services Administration, 1997).

The Johns Hopkins HIV Care Program, like most urban health care centers, treats large numbers of people with HIV infection or AIDS who have multiple comorbidities and complicated health care and enabling needs. They have had time to examine the process of transition to managed care and have concluded that the learning curve is steep, especially for academic health centers; that planning and implementing managed care takes time and requires a dedicated project director; and that although cost reduction is a clear goal, the key to success is proper risk adjustment and rate setting (Bartlett, 1998).

Tennessee's model differs from Maryland's in a few important ways. Tennessee relies on risk pools instead of risk adjustment, plans participate voluntarily both in subcontracting and in following treatment protocols, and plans use a coordinator to link medical and enabling services rather than carving out these services.

Homeless People

Homeless people provide an example of a socially dislocated population with extraordinary health care access barriers that require special outreach programs. Because of their extreme poverty, homeless people undoubtedly qualify for public benefit programs but frequently have difficulty applying for and accessing such programs (Burt, 1992; Rossi, 1989). Homeless people illustrate the convergence of several important factors including stigma, extreme poverty, the presence of complex medical and social needs, and a population that is difficult to track. The homeless use costly hospital and emergency services for care and can present a public health risk.

According to the U.S. Department of Housing and Urban Development, as many as 7 million Americans, 15 percent of whom are children, experienced being homeless at least once in the late 1980s, and in 1994, as many as 600,000 people in the U.S. were homeless on a given night. The population may have grown since the enactment of welfare reforms in 1996, which have limited access to public assistance (State Health Notes, 1998).

On any given night one-third to one-half of the estimated 600,000 homeless people will be adults with serious mental illness and/or substance abuse, and others will have HIV infection or AIDS and resurgent tuberculosis problems (Burt and Cohen, 1989; U.S. Department of Health and Human Services, 1992; U.S. Department of Housing and Urban Development, 1994). Such illnesses carry a real public health threat, which only compounds the stigma already associated with such disorders and with homelessness itself. Studies have shown that homeless people (in particular, those with SMIs and women) are more likely to be criminally victimized and that such victimization leads to a cycle of homelessness and repeated victimization, as well as episodic admissions to hospital emergency and acute care units (Caton et al., 1995; Lam and Rosenheck, 1998; U.S. Department of Housing and Urban Development, 1994).

Compared with nonhomeless people, homeless people (1) have a greater need for psychiatric emergency and inpatient services (Dickey et al., 1996; Rosenheck and Seibyl, 1998; Wuerker and Keenan, 1997); (2) have more hospital emergency department and inpatient admissions and longer lengths of stay attributable to substance abuse, mental illness, trauma, and respiratory, skin, and infectious disorders (Salit et al., 1998); and (3) use more high-cost services. In nearly all cases, inpatient admissions could have been prevented by earlier intervention and ongoing health maintenance activities.

Like other special-needs populations, homeless people attract categorical funding streams from both the private and public sectors. Local independent not-for-profit organizations and the faith community took the early lead in providing emergency services, including temporary shelter, food, and health services. Most states have relied on these efforts and modest state funding (only 27 states reported any special assistance [less than $5 million each] in 1991) for targeted services to the homeless population. The federal government started to fill the gap in the early 1980s with appropriations for the Emergency Food and Shelter Program, designed to combine federal funds with state and local not-for-profit organization resources to provide emergency assistance to the homeless population, and the Temporary Emergency Food Assistance Program. Other assistance came from the Emergency Assistance Program of the U.S. Department of Health and Human Services, and the Community Development Block Grant Program for which emergency services and shelters were eligible (U.S. Department of Housing and Urban Development, 1994).

The passage of the 1987 Stewart B. McKinney Homeless Assistance Act increased the federal government's role in addressing homelessness. More than 20 McKinney Act grant assistance programs fund the provision of emergency food and shelter, surplus goods, transitional housing, supportive housing, primary health care services, mental health care, alcohol and drug abuse treatment, education, and job training (U.S. Department of Housing and Urban Development, 1994).

Public hospitals, community health centers, and facilities for veterans have been the traditional safety net providers for the homeless population, but the categorical funding streams noted above have broadened the safety net considerably to include a wide range of private not-for-profit agencies in churches and other nontraditional settings.

Successful programs have integrated primary care services (medical, dental, and behavioral health care services) combined with case management, enabling services (such as transportation), and street and shelter outreach and have effectively created teams of registered nurses, nurse practitioners, primary care physicians, psychiatrists, dentists, case managers, outreach workers (for enrollment as well as engagement and retention), and social workers.

The Wasatch Homeless Health Care in Salt Lake City, Utah, is located across from a park where homeless people congregate and sees about 6,500 homeless individuals each year for a total of about 22,000 "office" visits. On-site services include primary care and pediatrics, dermatology, podiatry, eye care, dental care, and physical therapy. In addition to its staff of 17, the clinic relies on about 30 physician volunteers, AmeriCorps members, and medical students who run a Saturday clinic.

The Providence Health Care for the Homeless project in Rhode Island also relies on a combination of paid and volunteer staff from a wide range of disciplines. It sees about 1,850 homeless people annually, for a total of approximately 4,500 encounters. A mobile medical van staffed by rotations of more than 100 physicians, nurses, and medical students is the main outreach vehicle. It makes rounds to area shelters and soup kitchens in the evening. In addition, the program operates a multiservice center for clients who need enabling services, a Saturday walk-in clinic staffed by volunteer physicians, a women's program staffed 1 day a week by nurse practitioners under an agreement with a local nursing college, and a dental clinic staffed with volunteer dentists. The project relies on two local hospitals to donate laboratory services for diagnostic work and has an agreement with a community mental health center for outreach and referrals (State Health Notes, 1998).

LESSONS LEARNED

It appears that special-needs populations are more alike than different. These populations present common challenges to managed care programs—challenges that must be systematically evaluated in the context of geography, resources, demographics, and the availability and accessibility of special-needs providers before a managed care plan can be designed and implemented. Although there is no single solution for people with special needs, some common areas must be addressed by every state, preferably before moving this group into managed care plans. Special-needs populations in the safety net are vulnerable, first, by virtue of their poverty and, second, by virtue of the chronic illness, disability, or social circumstances that place them at increased risk of falling through the safety net. Early experience has suggested that slow and cautious movement toward managed care is the wisest approach to special-needs populations and that moving too quickly with insufficient planning can compromise the safety net for special-needs populations and can place consumers at risk.

The lessons that have been learned from this analysis fall into four areas: (1) problems of definition and data, (2) the service requirements of special-needs populations, (3) issues of costs and financing, and (4) the unique role of the consumer advocacy community.

Definitions and Data

Rates of disability vary from state to state, as do definitions of special needs. These variations lead to meaningful differences in treatment standards and the inclusion or exclusion of covered services in managed care contracts; they make it particularly difficult to track special-needs populations. Special longitudinal studies that are national in scope could provide a baseline from which states, managed care organizations, and providers could tailor their own data elements and studies to better plan, implement, and evaluate the services that they provide to special-needs populations. State consensus panels that involve all stakeholders might be convened to address the issue of definitions to better predict service need, utilization patterns, and costs.

Service Requirements of Special-Needs Populations

People with disabilities and chronic illnesses use a wide spectrum of health and enabling services, and service requirements can vary considerably among individuals and by diagnostic and disability group. Although many states have medical necessity laws that mandate the inclusion of such services, many managed care organizations interpret medical necessity more narrowly. For some groups, the provision of medical and enabling services is necessary but not sufficient. Those who are socially dislocated, such as homeless people or immigrants, require active, specially tailored outreach services. Thus, states should include specific language in contracts to protect consumer access to outreach as well as medical and enabling services. In most instances, such services have been and should continue to be provided by safety net providers.

In addition, although special-needs consumers require access to both primary and specialty care providers, little evidence suggests that the primary and specialty care safety nets are well coordinated. Single-point accountability services, such as case management and care coordinators, provide the glue for an otherwise fragmented system of care, and such services must be factored into the costs of service delivery. Finally, plans need to be flexible in defining the primary care providers for these patients.

Costs and Financing

The states vary widely in coverage and payment mechanisms for special-needs populations; this variation is so wide that for some conditions, like HIV infection and AIDS, the best predictor of care and outcomes is the state in which one lives. Rapidly evolving treatment standards for some special-needs populations render the use of retrospective cost methodologies ineffective for projecting future costs and payments. Carve-out and stand-alone models have dominated the market for the special-needs population, creating multiple tiers of coverage, responsibility, and accountability, and require new incentives to ensure appropriate service delivery. Thus, financing (e.g., health-based and service-based rate adjustment and risk pools), contracting, and regulatory mechanisms are critical ingredients to successful managed care plans for the special-needs population.

The Unique Role of Advocacy

It was apparent during the committee's site visits that consumer advocates, in particular those who represent populations with special needs, have begun to secure an important place in policy making related to managed care. Advocacy is an important factor in shaping health policy for special-needs populations. Each special-needs group reviewed in this chapter has a strong advocacy base that has been successful in marshaling scarce resources for their constituents' needs. They have won hard-fought legislative and regulatory battles that have improved access to and parity in care. In addition, they have contributed to the ongoing discourse about outcomes evaluation, quality, and effectiveness, with particular emphasis on measures more sensitive to special-needs populations, better consumer education on managed care, and better provider education on special needs. They have argued effectively that consumers and consumer needs must be represented in the managed care planning process and that contracts must include a comprehensive array of medically necessary services.

Sometimes a narrow advocacy focus can result in overly detailed rules that become counterproductive to the implementation of care and a burden to safety net providers that wish to serve special-needs consumers. Although advocates might find it difficult to move beyond the narrow boundaries of their particular special-needs constituency to the more inclusive boundaries of special needs in general, managed care will likely demand such a broadening of views. Advocates and consumers will be key players in the search for commonality among special-needs groups and in identifying meaningful differences that must be accommodated through variations in financing, contracting, or service delivery mechanisms and should be included as essential stakeholders at all stages of implementation of managed care plans.

GENERALIZATIONS TO THE LARGER SAFETY NET SYSTEM

Many of the lessons that have been learned and described in this chapter can and should be generalized to the entire safety net system. Although those with special needs served by the safety net system may be at higher risk and require the bundling of more services than others served by the safety net system, they provide a paradigm for the entire safety net population. For example, the need for comparable data systems that cross community and state lines is equally acute whether they are for people with HIV infection or AIDS or poor, uninsured, inner-city mothers. States must have meaningful data to maintain their authority and contractual obligations to the populations served by the safety net system. Similarly, the experiences with special-needs populations underscore the need for specific language in contract agreements as states undertake enrollment of safety net populations in managed care plans. The experiences with special needs populations certainly provide evidence that financing, contracting, and regulatory mechanisms are essential ingredients in any managed care plan involving safety net populations. Perhaps most important, this brief examination of special-needs populations emphasizes what many have long known: primary care and specialty care services in the safety net system remain fragmented and uncoordinated. As more of those served by the safety net system, particularly those who require coordinated or integrated services, are moved into managed care arrangements, the problems associated with fragmentation will become more acute and will demand solutions such as single-point accountability, point-of-service, care coordination, and case management. The committee believes that special-needs populations are the sentinels, and are signaling the effects for all Medicaid and uninsured people. They warrant continued study as an important barometer of the health of the safety net in the evolving health care marketplace.

REFERENCES

Alliance for Health Reform. 1998. *Managed Care and Vulnerable Americans: Mental Health Coverage.* Washington, DC: Alliance for Health Reform.

Alliance for Health Reform. 1997. *Managed Care and Vulnerable Americans: Children with Special Health Care Needs.* Washington, DC: Alliance for Health Reform.

Bartlett, J.G. 1998. Johns Hopkins University School of Medicine Medicaid AIDS Capitated Care Program. In: *Capitation of AIDS Treatment: The Health Resources and Services Administration SPNS Program Grantees.* Special Projects of National Significance Program, Health Resources and Services Administration. Washington, DC: U.S. Department of Health and Human Services.

Bartlett, J.G., and Moore, R.D. 1996. Are Protease Inhibitors Cost Effective? *The Hopkins HIV Report, 8*, 1, 6.

Bishop, C.E., and Skwara, K.C. 1997. *Medicaid Spending for Persons with Disabilities: Dimensions and Growth.* Waltham, MA: The Center for Vulnerable Populations, Brandeis University.

Blancquaert, I.R., Zvagulis, I., Gray-Donald, K., and Pless, I.B. 1992. Referral Patterns for Children with Chronic Diseases. *Pediatrics, 90*(1), 71–74.

Bozzette, S.A., Berry, S.H., Duan, N., Frankel, M.R., Leibowitz, A.A., Lefkowitz, D., Emmons, C., Senterfitt, J.W., Berk, M.L., Morton, S.C., and Shapiro, M.F. 1998. The Care of HIV-Infected Adults in the United States. *New England Journal of Medicine, 339*(26), 1897–1904.

Buchanan, R.J., and Smith, S.R. 1998. State Implementation of the AIDS Drug Assistance Programs. *Health Care Financing Review, 19*(3), 39–62.

Burt, M. 1992. *Over the Edge.* New York, NY: Russell Sage.

Burt, M., and Cohen, B. 1989. *America's Homeless: Numbers, Characteristics and the Programs that Serve Them.* Washington, DC: The Urban Institute.

Butler, P. 1993. *The Role of the Public Delivery System in a Universal Health Care Financing Program.* Background paper. Providing Care to the Poor, A Workshop on the Role of Public Providers. Washington, DC: The Henry J. Kaiser Family Foundation.

Caton, C.L., Shrout, P.E., Boanerges, D., Eagle, P.F., Opler, L.A., and Cournos, F. 1995. Risk Factors for Homelessness Among Women with Schizophrenia. *American Journal of Public Health, 85*(8), 1153–1156.

Centers for Disease Control and Prevention. 1997. *HIV/AIDS Surveillance Report: U.S. HIV and AIDS Cases Reported Through June 1997*, Midyear Edition, Vol. 9, No. 1. Atlanta, GA: Centers for Disease Control and Prevention.

Chang, C.F., Kiser, L.J., Bailey, J.E., Martins, M., Gibson, W.C., Schaberg, K.A., Mirvis, D.M., and Applegate, W.B. 1998. Tennessee's Failed Managed Care Program for Mental Health and Substance Abuse Services. *JAMA, 279*(11), 864–869.

Dickey, B., Gonzalez, O., Latimer, E., Powers, K., Schutt, R., and Goldfinger, S. 1996. Use of Mental Health Services by Formerly Homeless Adults Residing in Group and Independent Housing. *Psychiatric Services, 47*(2), 152–158.

Fasciano, N.J., Cherlow, A.L., Turner, B.J., and Thornton, C.V. 1998. Profile of Medicare Beneficiaries with AIDS: Application of an AIDS Casefinding Algorithm. *Health Care Financing Review, 19*(3), 19–38.

Foster, S., Gregory, A., Niederhausen, P., Rapallo, D., and Westmoreland, T. 1999. *Federal HIV/AIDS Spending: A Budget Chartbook*. Menlo Park, CA: The Henry J. Kaiser Family Foundation.

Health Resources and Services Administration. 1997. *HIV Capitation Risk Adjustment Conference Report*. Washington, DC: Office of Science and Epidemiology, HIV/AIDS Bureau, Center for Managed Care, Health Resources and Services Administration, U.S. Department of Health and Human Services.

Hellinger, F.J. 1998. Cost and Financing of Care for Persons with HIV Disease: An Overview. *Health Care Financing Review, 19*(3), 5–18.

Hirschel, B., and Francioli, P. 1998. Progress and Problems in the Fight Against AIDS. *New England Journal of Medicine, 338*(13), 906–908.

Institute of Medicine. 1996. *Paying Attention to Children in a Changing Health Care System*. Washington, DC: National Academy Press.

Institute of Medicine. 1997. *Managing Managed Care*. Washington, DC: National Academy Press.

Institute of Medicine. 1998. *America's Children: Health Insurance and Access to Care*. Washington, DC: National Academy Press.

Ireys, H.T., Grason, H.A., and Guyer, B. 1996. Assuring Quality of Care for Children with Special Needs in Managed Care Organizations: Roles for Pediatricians. *Pediatrics, 98*(2), 178–185.

Johns Hopkins University. 1997. *Clinicians Guide. The Johns Hopkins University ACG Case-Mix Adjustment System*, version 4.0. Baltimore, MD: Johns Hopkins University.

The Kaiser Commission on Medicaid and the Uninsured. 1999. *Medicaid Facts: Medicaid's Disabled Population and Managed Care*. Washington, DC: The Henry J. Kaiser Family Foundation.

The Kaiser Commission on the Future of Medicaid. 1996. *Medicaid's Role for Persons with HIV/AIDS*. Washington, DC: The Henry J. Kaiser Family Foundation.

Kaye, N., Pernice, C., and Pelletier, H. 1999. *Medicaid Managed Care: A Guide for States*. 4th ed. Portland, ME: National Academy for State Health Policy.

Kuhlthau, K., Walker, D.K., Perrin, J.M., Bauman, L., Gortmaker, S.L., Newacheck, P.W., and Stein, R.E.K. 1998. Assessing Managed Care for Children with Chronic Conditions. *Health Affairs, 17*(4), 42–52.

Lam, J., and Rosenheck, R. 1998. The Effect of Victimization on Clinical Outcomes of Homeless Persons with Serious Mental Illness. *Psychiatric Services, 49*(5), 678–683.

LaPlante, M.P. 1991. The Demographics of Disability. *The Millbank Quarterly, 2*(55), 55–77.

LaPlante, M.P., Rice, D.P., and Cyril, J.K. 1993. Health Insurance Coverage of People with Disabilities in the U.S., pp. 1–6. In: *Disability Statistics Abstract*, No. 7. Washington, DC: National Institute on Disability and Rehabilitation Research, U.S. Department of Education.

Liptak, G.S., and Revell, G.M. 1989. Community Physician's Role in Case Management of Children with Chronic Illnesses. *Pediatrics, 84*(3), 465–471.

Liska, D. 1997. *Medicaid Overview: A Complex Program.* Washington, DC: The Urban Institute.

McPherson, M., Arango, P., Fox, H., Lauver, C., McManus, M., Newacheck, P.W., Perrin, J.M., Shonkoff, J.P., and Strickland, B. 1998. A New Definition of Children with Special Health Care Needs. *Pediatrics, 102*(1), 137–140.

Mechanic, D. 1998. Emerging Trends in Mental Health Policy and Practice. *Health Affairs, 17*(6), 82–98.

Moore, R.D., and Bartlett, J.G. 1996. Combination Antiretroviral Therapy in HIV Infection, an Economic Perspective. *PharmacoEconomics, 2,* 109–113.

National Governors' Association. 1996. *Serving Children with Special Health Care Needs Within Medicaid Managed Care.* Washington, DC: National Governors' Association.

Neff, J.M., and Anderson, G. 1995. Protecting Children with Chronic Illness in a Competitive Marketplace. *JAMA, 274*(23), 1866–1869.

Newacheck, P.W., and Taylor, W.R. 1992. Childhood Chronic Illness: Prevalence, Severity, and Impact. *American Journal of Public Health, 82,* 364–371.

Pine, P.L. 1998. Overview. *Health Care Financing Review, 19*(3), 1–3.

Rawlings-Sekunda, J., and Kaye, N. 1998. *Emerging Practices and Policy in Medicaid Managed Care for People with HIV/AIDS: Case Studies of Six Programs.* Portland, ME: National Academy for State Health Policy.

Regenstein, M., and Schroer, C. 1998. *Medicaid Managed Care for Persons with Disabilities: State Profiles.* Washington, DC: The Henry J. Kaiser Family Foundation.

Rosenbaum, S., Shin, P., Zakheim, M., Shaw, K., and Teitelbaum, J. 1998. *Negotiating the New Health System: A Nationwide Study of Medicaid Managed Care Contracts. Special Report: Mental Illness and Addiction Disorder Treatment and Prevention.* Washington, DC: Center for Health Services Policy and Research, The George Washington University.

Rosenheck, R., and Seibyl, C.L. 1998. Homelessness, Health Service Use and Related Costs. *Medical Care, 36*(8), 1256–1264.

Rossi, P.H. 1989. *Down and Out in America.* Chicago, IL: University of Chicago Press.

Salit, S., Kuhn, E.M., Hartz, A.J., Vu, J.M., and Mosso, A.L. 1998. Hospitalization Costs Associated with Homelessness in New York City. *New England Journal of Medicine, 338*(24), 1734–1740.

Schlesinger, M., and Mechanic, D. 1993. Challenges for Managed Competition from Chronic Illness. *Health Affairs Supplement, 12,* 123–137.

Somers, S.A., and Brodsky, K.L. 1997. A Health Care System in Transformation: Making It Work for People with Chronic Health and Social Problems. *Health Strategies Quarterly.* Princeton, NJ: Center for Health Care Strategies.

State Health Notes. 1998. Health Care for the Homeless: Reaching Out to Streets, Shelters. *State Health Notes, 19*(289), 1–2.

Substance Abuse and Mental Health Services Administration Managed Care Tracking System. 1998. *State Profiles on Public Sector Managed Behavioral Healthcare and Other Reforms.* Fairfax, VA: The Lewin Group.

Trupin, L., Rice, D.P., and Max, W. 1995. Who Pays for the Medical Care of People with Disabilities?, pp. 1–4. In: *Disability Statistics Abstract,* No. 13. Washington, DC: National Institute on Disability and Rehabilitation Research, U.S. Department of Education.

U.S. Department of Health and Human Services. 1992. *State and Local Perspectives on the McKinney Act.* Washington, DC: Office of the Inspector General, U.S. Department of Health and Human Services.

U.S. Department of Housing and Urban Development. 1994. *Priority: Home! The Federal Plan to Break the Cycle of Homelessness.* Publication HUD-1451-CPD (1). Washington, DC: U.S. Department of Housing and Urban Development.

Wenger, B.L., Kaye, H.S., and LaPlante, M. 1997. Disabilities Among Children, pp. 1–6. *In: Disability Statistics Abstract*, No. 15. Washington, DC: National Institute of Disability and Rehabilitation Research, U.S. Department of Education.

Wuerker, A.K., and Keenan, C.K. 1997. Patterns of Psychiatric Service Use by Homeless Mentally Ill Clients. *Psychiatric Quarterly, 68*(2), 101–116.

Young, P.C., and Schork, S.Y. 1994. The Role of the Primary Care Physician in the Care of Children with Serious Heart Disease. *Pediatrics, 94*(3), 284–290.

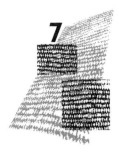

7

Findings and Recommendations

The committee believes that the first priority of any national health care policy should be to ensure that each individual has access to needed health care services. In the absence of comprehensive health care coverage, the United States has relied on a set of loosely organized community-based safety net providers to address the health care needs of the uninsured and other populations. The collapse of the safety net in a community may require this population to face formidable barriers to obtaining the health care that they need. The health care safety net has historically functioned in a precarious fiscal environment, suffering through many changes in the national and local economies, changes in public policies, changes in the health care market, and changes in funding sources. Despite today's robust economy, safety net providers—especially core safety net providers—are being buffeted by the cumulative and concurrent effects of major health policy and market changes. The convergence and potentially adverse consequences of these new and powerful dynamics leads the committee to be highly concerned about the future viability of the safety net. Although safety net providers have proven to be both resilient and resourceful, the committee believes that many providers may be unable to survive the current environment. Taken alone, the growth in Medicaid managed care enrollment; the retrenchment or elimination of key direct and indirect subsidies that providers have relied upon to help finance uncompensated care; and the continued growth in the number of uninsured people would make it difficult for many safety net providers to survive. Taken together, these trends are beginning to place unparalleled strain on the health care safety net in many parts of the country.

In most communities the core safety net has continued to survive and to respond to the new requirements of managed care, but its underlying structure and long-term viability are increasingly threatened. The consequences of looming cuts in disproportionate share hospital (DSH) payments and the elimination of cost-based reimbursement for federally qualified health centers (FQHCs) have not yet been fully felt. Adding to these mounting pressures is new evidence that private providers and institutions operating in more advanced managed care markets have become less able or less willing to maintain their past commitments to the provision of uncompensated care. Cuts in the Medicare program and other related consequences of the Balanced Budget Act of 1997 (BBA) may further reduce the capacities of these providers to continue to provide service to the uninsured population, adding to the burden of the core safety net.

Ironically, these developments and retrenchments are taking place against the backdrop of a strong economy, a low rate of inflation in health care costs, and budget surpluses at the federal, state, and local levels. At the same time, however, significant increases in health insurance premiums and the number of uninsured adults are projected. Any downturn in the economy will further degrade the increasingly tenuous safety net system. The committee believes that the effects of these combined forces and dynamics demand the immediate attention of public policy officials and recommends a series of actions to help ensure the continued viability of a core health care safety net for the nation's most vulnerable populations.

FINDINGS

Finding 1. The shift to Medicaid managed care can have adverse effects on core safety net providers and the uninsured and other vulnerable populations who rely on them for care. These dynamics demand greater attention and scrutiny by policy leaders and administrative agencies at the federal, state, and local levels.

The growth in price competition and the reduced payments made by private payers has made Medicaid a more attractive payer in many communities. Providers that previously shunned this market because of low reimbursement rates are now competing for Medicaid patients, especially with the introduction of managed care. The committee heard evidence that in some communities these developments have had the positive effect of offering beneficiaries a broader network of providers from which to choose. Enhanced choice of quality providers is desirable as a matter of equity and fairness and can create needed incentives for all providers to improve their performance and be more responsive to patients.

The committee is concerned, however, that programs that promote choice are not always implemented in a manner that adequately

- considers the impact on the ability of core safety net providers to sustain their missions to provide care for indigent populations,
- ensures that patients are adequately informed about their choices and that those choices are facilitated,
- ensures that patients who require complex coordinated care are supported by the necessary enabling services, and
- ensures that continuity of care is not seriously disrupted as patients cycle on and off Medicaid and plans enter and exit the Medicaid managed care market.

Given the special characteristics of the Medicaid population, the committee heard and read testimony suggesting that expanded choice could hold unintended risks for beneficiaries and those who provide care for indigent populations. For example:

- The categorical and episodic nature of Medicaid eligibility means that individuals tend to cycle off and on coverage, often with long spells without insurance. Most managed care organizations and their providers, especially those new to the Medicaid market, often have no formal responsibility or mission to take care of patients when they become uninsured. These new dynamics can impair continuity of care for patients who may have switched from a provider who will serve them whether or not they have Medicaid coverage to a provider who can only serve them when they are receiving Medicaid benefits. The dynamics can also undermine the stability of a community's safety net if core safety net providers lose their Medicaid patient base and other safety net providers find it difficult to shift the costs for additional uninsured patients in a increasingly competitive environment.
- Although Medicaid was not originally intended to support care for the uninsured population, over the years Medicaid revenues have come to provide a critical "silent subsidy" that helps core safety net providers pay for fixed infrastructure costs, freeing limited grant funds and other revenues to pay for care for uninsured patients. Thus, care for Medicaid and uninsured patients became inexorably linked, creating an interdependency in the absence of more explicit state or federal subsidies and policies regarding care for the uninsured population. The increasing separation of care for Medicaid beneficiaries and care for the growing number

of uninsured individuals may have the effect of destabilizing the safety net in many communities.

• A number of states have been successful in encouraging commercial and other plans to enter the Medicaid market by creating a hospitable market environment and offering attractive premium rates. Recently, however, a number of major commercial plans have exited all or major parts of the market because of the complexities of serving Medicaid patients, the inability to make a profit, and administrative requirements that they perceive to be burdensome. These developments have spurred the growth of Medicaid-only plans, which are organized in many cases by local safety net providers. Thus, safety net providers are once again providing care for their traditional patient populations, but often with fewer overall resources, more administrative requirements, and an increased demand for uncompensated care.

Finding 2. Managed care principles offer significant potential for improved health care for Medicaid patients, but implementation problems can undermine this potential.

The literature holds convincing evidence on the potential of managed care principles to improve the quality and efficiency of care for most patients and accountability to patients. When properly implemented, managed care can (1) promote comprehensive, integrated care with an emphasis on primary care, prevention, and population health; (2) offer greater incentives for efficient and appropriate care; and (3) provide a greater accountability for performance on the part of providers.

In addition, the growth of competition and choice in an environment of Medicaid managed care has produced new and powerful incentives for safety net providers to raise the bar in areas of operating efficiency, administrative and information systems, customer service, and general accountability to patients and payers. Safety net providers operating in a managed care environment may be able to offer vulnerable populations additional benefits in the important enabling, social, and outreach services that many of these patients require.

Despite this potential, however, the committee collected substantial evidence that raises the following concerns:

• The health plans and providers that serve Medicaid beneficiaries may have conflicting incentives that can diminish the potential value of managed care. For example, since poor patients tend to go on and off Medicaid, some health plans may see little advantage in investing in preventive care or other services to improve the long-term health of their Medicaid members.

- To remain viable a number of community-based providers are creating joint ventures with large hospitals or academic health center-owned systems. For example, many safety net providers do not have sufficient capital to invest in the management information systems and other capital improvements necessary to succeed in managed care. Although affiliations with a hospital or an academic health center may hold significant advantages, these uneven partnerships, if not properly structured, could affect the long-term ability of community-based safety net providers to maintain their past commitments to the uninsured population.
- Inadequate capitation rates in many states and the absence of adequate risk-adjustment tools may be forcing many safety net providers to assume substantial financial risk without sufficient reserves or other protections against insolvency.

The transition of state Medicaid programs from bill payer to prudent purchaser requires the development of specific new skills by program administrators, including skills in contracting, premium rate setting, quality and financial oversight, patient education, and enrollment protocols. The committee finds that in many states the implementation of managed care has been attempted with insufficient preparation and staffing. Although some states have moved to managed care to improve access and quality of care, in recent years, a priority objective for most states appears to be program cost savings.

The committee finds it difficult to gauge the success of the states' Medicaid managed care initiatives. Results have been inconsistent and vary widely from state to state. The committee found that better methods are needed to both capture and disseminate the lessons that have been learned and the problems that need to be avoided, as well as to help diminish inappropriate and potentially harmful interstate variations in the provision of safety net services.

> **Finding 3**. The financial viability of core safety net providers is even more at risk today than in the past because of the combined effects of three major dynamics: (1) the rising number of uninsured individuals; (2) the full impact of mandated Medicaid managed care in a more competitive health care marketplace; and (3) the erosion and uncertainty of major direct and indirect subsidies that have helped support safety net functions.

Safety net providers have always operated in a precarious financial environment and over the years have learned to survive in both good and bad economic times. The committee believes that, absent new policies, the increasing demand for care for indigent populations, the diminishing resources to support such care, and the mounting access barriers faced by uninsured people will endanger the fragile patchwork of providers and institutions that serve this nation's most vulnerable groups.

> **Finding 4.** The patchwork organization and the patchwork funding of the safety net vary widely from community to community, and the availability of care for the uninsured and other vulnerable populations increasingly depends on where they live.

Although federal Medicare, Medicaid, and other policies (such as cost-based reimbursement for FQHCs) have a critical impact on the financial viability of the safety net system, the strength and viability of a community's safety net system are highly dependent on state and local support, state Medicaid policies, the structure of the local health care marketplace, and the economic health of the community. With the devolution of responsibilities from the federal government to state and local governments, care for vulnerable populations is increasingly determined by local economic, political, and social factors. These trends are resulting in ever widening state and community variations in care for vulnerable populations and the adequacy of the health care safety net.

The committee found substantial evidence that states with the greatest demands for safety net services often have the weakest economic, political, and social infrastructures to effectively respond to local needs.

Although policies of devolution have contributed to innovative programs and policies directed to care for vulnerable populations, they have also made it more difficult to collect adequate and comparable data to track and monitor the changing status of state and local safety net organizations and how program and policy changes are affecting care for vulnerable populations.

> **Finding 5.** The committee found that most safety net providers have thus far been able to adapt to the changing environment. Even for these providers, however, the stresses of these changes have made it increasingly difficult for them to maintain their missions while protecting their financial margins. In addition, the full consequences of changing market forces, increases in the number of uninsured, and reduced levels of reimbursement have not yet been felt by these providers in some communities. The committee further observed that the current capacity for monitoring the status of safety net providers is inadequate for providing timely and systematic evidence about the effects of these forces.

Although the committee heard frequent testimony and studied a number of reports about the negative consequences of the various changes in the environment of safety net providers, it was continuously frustrated by its inability to find a single source where such information was collected and analyzed. It was also evident that the information that was available took many years to assemble and that important data was often missing or only describing the situation in a few communities.

In some parts of the country, all of the major forces of change, including growth in the numbers of uninsured individuals, high rates of penetration of mandated Medicaid managed care, strong market competition, and the full impact of the BBA of 1997, have not yet converged, making it possible for many core safety net providers to maintain their missions to provide care for the uninsured population. The committee believes, however, that in the current policy and political environment, these forces will continue to have increasingly adverse effects.

Safety net providers are placing major emphases on gaining contracts with managed care organizations, developing partnerships and networks to gain leverage and to benefit from economies of scale, diversifying funding streams, improving clinical and administrative protocols, and improving customer-oriented services.

- Virtually all safety net providers have come to realize that they must participate in Medicaid managed care, but little is known about what adaptive strategies appear to be the most successful.
- Although on the whole the safety net has remained intact, many of these organizations are becoming increasingly fragile given the growing number of uninsured individuals and cutbacks in grants and revenues. New studies show that managed care cost pressures are forcing other providers to retrench on the provision of care for vulnerable populations, placing an even greater burden on the core safety net.
- State and local policies and programs that support care for vulnerable populations have proved to be critically important to the ability of community safety net systems to remain viable while maintaining their missions to provide care for the uninsured population.
- At this stage of Medicaid managed care and restructuring of the U.S. health care system, few reliable and consistent data exist to determine clearly how beneficiaries are faring in the new environment.

The patchwork and categorical nature of funding for the safety net has created barriers to systems building, integration, and more flexible responses to new requirements, all of which are critical for successful adaptation to managed care. Safety net organizations are not well integrated at the regional or local level. There are only a few examples of communities in which core safety net providers have integrated into a more seamless system (e.g., Denver Health and Cambridge Hospital in Massachusetts). In most cases, community health centers, public hospitals, and public health departments do not have common governance, shared physical or information infrastructures, joint staffs, common patient identifiers, or defined integration of services. The historical separation of funding streams as well as the different missions and constituencies of various providers have worked against effective collaboration.

A resurgence of inflation in health care costs, an economic downturn, or further increases in the rolls of the uninsured could further destabilize the safety net and place essential care for America's vulnerable populations at the risk of significant peril. In light of these circumstances, the committee finds a compelling need for a stronger ongoing capacity to monitor the changing status of the safety net.

RECOMMENDATIONS

Recommendation 1. Federal and state policy makers should explicitly take into account and address the full impact (both intended and unintended) of changes in Medicaid policies on the viability of safety net providers and the populations they serve.

In making this recommendation, the committee believes that the following issues need heightened public policy attention:

• failure to take into consideration the impact on safety net providers of changes in Medicaid policy could have a significant negative effect on the ability of these providers to continue their mission to serve the uninsured population, particularly those who move back and forth between being eligible for Medicaid and being uninsured;
• the adequacy and fairness of Medicaid managed care rates;
• the erosion of the Medicaid patient base and the financial stability of core safety net providers that must continue to care for the uninsured population;
• the declining ability or willingness of non-core safety net providers to provide care for the uninsured population; and
• the current instability of the Medicaid managed care market including the rapid entry and exit of plans and the impact of this churning of program beneficiaries.

Recommendation 2. All federal programs and policies targeted to support the safety net and the populations it serves should be reviewed for their effectiveness in meeting the needs of the uninsured.

Major new forces have altered the financing and delivery of health care services, including the move to managed care by both private and public payers, the separation of care for Medicaid patients from care for uninsured individuals, the erosion and retrenchment of direct and indirect subsidies that have helped provide care for those without coverage, and the increasing concentration of care for the uninsured population among fewer providers. These dynamics call for a careful review of programs and policies that were designed to improve access to care for vulnerable populations and support the providers that serve them to make sure that these programs are still effectively targeted to meet their original objectives. The committee believes that such an analysis is especially important given the growing number of uninsured Americans and the declining ability to meet their health care needs. Federal health care programs that provide direct or indirect support for safety net providers and for services for vulnerable populations should be reviewed and modified to ensure that any funding allocation formula specifies explicit criteria for the delivery of services to the uninsured population as a basis for support. Eligibility for Medicaid and Medicare DSH funds should also be reexamined to include a greater focus on the level and share of services for the uninsured. Although the committee believes strongly that no funds should be diverted from the core safety net, any funds that become available as a result of this reexamination should be distributed in a manner that ensures that providers of both ambulatory and inpatient care are eligible to receive support.

> **Recommendation 3. The committee recommends that concerted efforts be directed to improving this nation's capacity and ability to monitor the changing structure, capacity, and financial stability of the safety net to meet the health care needs of the uninsured and other vulnerable populations.**

The committee believes that the fragility of local safety nets has the potential to become a national crisis, and therefore, it calls for stronger federal tracking, direction, and targeted direct support. At this time, no single entity in the federal government has the responsibility for monitoring and tracking the status of America's health care safety net and its ability to meet the needs of those who rely on its services. Various agencies have responsibility for programs and policies that affect one part of the safety net delivery system (e.g., the Health Resources and Services Administration, the Centers for Disease Control and Prevention, the Substance Abuse and Mental Health Services Administration, the Health Care Financing Administration, the Head Start program, the Indian Health

Service, and the Departments of Veterans Affairs, Defense, Agriculture, and Housing and Urban Development), but no comprehensive, coordinated tracking and reporting capability exists. Although it acknowledges the appropriate roles and responsibilities of the various agencies and the benefits of state and local innovations, the committee believes that such a tracking capability could promote public accountability, as well as a more coordinated approach to data collection, technical assistance, and the application and dissemination of best practices.

A number of organizational settings could be considered for the placement of an enhanced safety net tracking and monitoring activity, including an existing agency, department, or program, or a newly established entity. Although the committee elected not to come to a final decision on where such an entity could be placed, it did discuss and identify the major organizational attributes that would be needed to enable a safety net oversight entity to successfully carry out its mission. The committee strongly believes that such an entity should be independent; organized as an ongoing activity with dedicated staff; nonpartisan in its membership; and include a range of expertise required to carry out its charge. Such an oversight body would affect a number of state and local entities and would cut across several federal agencies. In identifying these attributes the committee viewed with favor an organization like the Medical Payment Advisory Commission (MedPAC) with its mandate to report directly to Congress. Alternatively, the oversight body could reside in the executive branch at a Departmental level. As an example of the executive branch model, the committee was impressed with the work and impact of the President's Advisory Commission on Consumer Protection and Quality in the Health Care Industry. However, the Quality Commission had a limited term, consistent with its mandate to produce recommendations for action and implementation by other parts of the federal government and the private sector. The committee's proposed tracking and monitoring activity would require an ongoing term of operation, since its major function would be to assess, monitor, and report on the status of America's health care safety net over time. The committee in its deliberations referred to the monitoring and oversight entity as the Safety Net Organizations and Patient Advisory Commission (SNOPAC).

To carry out its mission, the committee recommends that the initial activities of a safety net oversight entity include the following:

- monitor the major safety net funding programs (e.g., Medicaid, the State Children's Health Insurance Program [SCHIP], Title V, FQHCs, and the various government DSH payment plans) to document and analyze the effects of changes in these programs on the safety net and the health of vulnerable populations;

- track the impact of the BBA of 1997 and other forces on the capacity of other key providers in the safety net system to continue their supportive roles in the core safety net system;
- monitor existing data sets to assess the status of the safety net and health outcomes for vulnerable populations;
- wherever possible, link and integrate the existing data systems to enhance their current ability and to track changes in the status of the safety net and health outcomes for vulnerable populations;
- support the development of new data systems where existing data are insufficient or inadequate;
- establish an early-warning system to identify impending failures of safety net systems and providers;
- provide accurate and timely information to federal, state, and local policy makers on the factors that led to the failures and the projected consequences of such failures;
- help monitor the transition of the population receiving Supplemental Security Income into Medicaid managed care including careful review of the degree to which safety net-based health plans have the capacity (e.g., case management and management information system infrastructure) to provide quality managed care services to this population and the degree to which these plans may be overburdened by adverse selection; and
- identify and disseminate best practices for more effective application of the lessons that have been learned.

> **Recommendation 4. Given the growing number of uninsured people, the adverse effects of Medicaid managed care on safety net provider revenues, and the absence of concerted public policies directed at increasing the rate of insurance coverage, the committee believes that a new targeted federal initiative should be established to help support core safety net providers that care for a disproportionate number of uninsured and other vulnerable people.**

Funding would be in the form of competitive three-year grants. Grants will vary in size, based on the scope of the project. Sources of financing could include funds available from the federal budget surplus and unspent funds from SCHIP and other insurance expansion programs. Although the committee projects such a new initiative may require a minimum of $2.5 billion ranging over five years, the specific size and scope of this program should be determined by the administration and the U.S. Congress and should be modified based on an assessment of the parameters of the problem by the safety net oversight entity. These assessments should be an ongoing responsibility of the safety net oversight entity.

The following principles should govern the distribution of these funds:

• Because the committee recognizes the challenges of delivering coordinated, seamless care for the poor uninsured and other vulnerable individuals at a time when the number of such people is increasing, the new initiative should concentrate on both the infrastructure for such care and subsidies of the care itself. Multiple models could be funded under this initiative, mirroring the multiple models of safety net arrangements in the various states and local communities. For example, in some areas a large safety net hospital could take the lead and join with other providers, including community-based clinics. A state or local government could stimulate cooperative efforts in other areas, participating with its own service-delivery capacity. In still others, coalitions of ambulatory care providers, such as community health centers allied with local private physicians, could form and undertake the initiative.

• Funds could be used for infrastructure improvements (e.g., for equipment, rehabilitation of unattractive and inefficient buildings, and management information systems) or to help defray costs or support items and activities such as legal and other costs related to establishment of the network (in ways to avoid charges of antitrust and fraud and abuse), improvements in quality of care (e.g., patient tracking systems, reengineering, and programs targeted to high-risk patients), and, where needed, the health care itself.

• Funds would be available to communities that demonstrate the potential capacity to deliver comprehensive services, to track patients and their outcomes as they move through the system, and to provide appropriate outreach and marketing efforts to reach patients with special needs. The allocations would specifically reward initiatives with demonstrated commitment and capacity to improve access and health outcomes for poor uninsured individuals in the community. Continuation of funding would be based upon ongoing satisfactory performance and accountability.

• Eligibility for funding would include a maintenance of effort requirement with documentation that the new funding would supplement and not replace state or local funding already directed to this effort.

During the time the committee was completing its study, the U.S. Department of Health and Human Services (DHHS), as part of its FY 2000 budget request, proposed a five year initiative designed to increase the capacity and effectiveness of the nation's health care safety net providers. To begin this effort, $25 million in the form of grant funding was appropriated under the FY 2000 Appropriations Act. The committee believes this new national program, the Community Access Program, which will provide funding for approximately 20 communities in the coming year, represents a good first step.

Recommendation 5. The committee recommends that technical assistance programs and policies targeted to improving the operations and competitive position of safety net providers be enhanced and better coordinated.

Several federal agencies including the Health Resources and Services Administration, the Health Care Financing Administration, the Substance Abuse and Mental Health Services Administration, and the Centers for Disease Control and Prevention currently provide technical assistance to some safety net providers, but these funds are usually targeted exclusively to the programs funded by the respective agencies. The committee strongly believes that technical assistance funds should promote capacity building and the management and operating capabilities of safety net providers seeking to compete in a managed care environment. Technical assistance programs should promote rather than deter the development of partnerships and collaborations that can contribute to these objectives.

The committee believes the following areas require specific attention:

• management of service delivery and implementation of changes, including improvements in management information systems, appointment scheduling systems, patient telephone access, efforts to streamline operations, and reengineering of services so that they are more responsive to patients;

• development of new business skills such as negotiating managed care contracts and developing marketing techniques to maintain and expand the patient base of safety net providers;

• development and collection of reliable data on which to calibrate rates and assign appropriate risks to develop appropriate reimbursement systems; and

• nonmedical factors that affect utilization and health outcomes of low-income and other vulnerable patients using the health care delivery system (e.g., care-seeking behavior, cultural competence, and public health interventions).

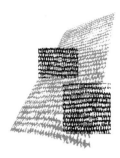

Appendixes

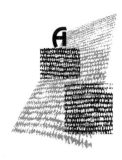

Committee Biographies

Stuart H. Altman, Ph.D. (*Chair*), Sol C. Chaikin Professor of National Health Policy at The Florence Heller Graduate School for Social Policy, Brandeis University, is an economist whose research interests are primarily in the area of federal health policy. He was appointed in December 1997 by President Clinton to the National Bipartisan Commission on the Future of Medicare. For 12 years he was chairman of the congressionally legislated Prospective Payment Assessment Commission responsible for advising Congress and the Administration on the Medicare Diagnostic Related Group Hospital Payment System and other system reforms. Dr. Altman is a member of the Institute of Medicine of the National Academy of Sciences, a member of the Board of Overseers of Beth Israel Deaconess Medical Center in Boston, Massachusetts, and chairman of the Board of the Institute for Health Policy at Brandeis University. He is chair of the Robert Wood Johnson Foundation sponsored Council on the Economic Impact of Health System Change, a private, nonpartisan group whose mission is to analyze important economic aspects of the U.S. health care system and evaluate proposed changes in the system. Dr. Altman has M.A. and Ph.D. degrees in economics from the University of California at Los Angeles and has taught at Brown University as well as the Graduate School of Public Policy, the University of California at Berkeley.

John G. Bartlett, M.D., is professor of medicine and chief of the Division of Infectious Diseases at Johns Hopkins University School of Medicine. Dr. Bartlett has been the principal investigator for $30 million in research funds at Hopkins and has written over 600 articles or chapters and 11 books (29 editions). His major interests are antibiotic-associated colitis, pneumonia, anaerobic infections, HIV infection and AIDS, and managed care. He received his M.D. from Upstate Medical Center in Syracuse in 1959 and completed training in internal medicine at Peter Bent Brigham in Boston, Massachusetts, and at the University of Alabama in Birmingham. His infectious disease fellowship was at the University of California at Los Angeles-Wadsworth Veterans Affairs Center in Los Angeles.

Raymond J. Baxter, Ph.D., is executive vice president at The Lewin Group in Falls Church, Virginia. He heads the firm's national public policy practice, and his consulting focuses on the areas of health systems reform, policy development, strategic planning, organizational design, and the management of change. He has worked with government and the private sector at the state, local, and national levels and has particular expertise in the areas of public health, mental health, long-term care, and HIV-related services. Dr. Baxter has over 20 years of experience in public health management, including service as the director of public health for San Francisco and the president of the New York City Health and Hospitals Corporation. Dr. Baxter holds a Ph.D. from the Woodrow Wilson School of Public and International Affairs, Princeton University.

John Billings, J.D., is currently an associate professor at the Robert F. Wagner Graduate School of Public Service at New York University, and he is the director of the school's Center for Health and Public Service Research. Previously, Mr. Billings was the principal investigator of a study for the Robert Wood Johnson Foundation and the United Hospital Fund of New York that involved analysis of patterns of hospital admission rates and emergency department utilization as tools to evaluate access barriers to outpatient care and to assess the performance of the ambulatory care delivery system. Mr. Billings is currently the principal investigator on a project funded by the Robert Wood Johnson Foundation to assess models for delivering primary care to low-income populations and is co-principal investigator in an effort with Columbia University and the United Hospital Fund of New York to evaluate the impact of Medicaid managed care in New York City. He has also worked extensively analyzing the problems of the medically indigent population and developing solutions for coverage and provision of care for the uninsured population. Mr. Billings is the former executive director of the John A. Hartford Foundation. Mr. Billings holds a law degree from the University of California at Berkeley.

Patricia A. Gabow, M.D., is chief executive officer and medical director of Denver Health and Hospital Systems. Dr. Gabow is also professor of medicine in the Division of Renal Disease at the University of Colorado School of Medicine. Her major research area is in polycystic kidney disease. She has authored more than 120 articles and book chapters. Dr. Gabow is a member of the executive committee and president-elect of the National Association of Public Hospitals and Health Systems and a member of the Board of the National Public Health and Hospital Institute. She received her M.D. degree from the University of Pennsylvania School of Medicine.

Mary L. Hennrich, M.S., is the chief executive officer of CareOregon Health Plan, Inc. Previous positions include director of the Primary Care and Health Systems Division, director of Field Services and Program Management Section, and director of Countywide Services in the Multnomah County Oregon Health Department. Her recent publications include *Successful Strategies for Managing Care in a Dynamic Market—Risk and Care Management for Special Populations* and *Collaboration to Improve Access and Create a Healthy Community—Oregon Health Systems in Collaboration: Lessons Learned from a Community Care Network Demonstration Site.* Ms. Hennrich received her M.S. in nursing at the University of Portland.

Sandral Hullett, M.D., M.P.H., is executive director of West Alabama Health Services, a community health center located in rural west Alabama. Her experience in research and grants include project director, School and Church Based Outreach Program, funded by the Robert Wood Johnson Foundation, and principal investigator, Antihypertensive and Lipid-Lowering Treatment to Prevent Heart Attack Trial, funded by the National Heart, Lung, and Blood Institute. Dr. Hullett has coauthored several publications, namely, *Alabama CHC Leads* and *Interdisciplinary Training Program, Interdisciplinary Health Care Training Program* (1993). Her educational background includes a bachelor's degree from Alabama A&M University, a medical degree from the Medical College of Pennsylvania, and a master's in public health from the University of Alabama.

Thomas G. Irons, M.D., is professor of pediatrics and associate vice chancellor for health sciences, East Carolina University School of Medicine. He also serves as president of HealthEast, a corporation formed by the School of Medicine and the Pitt County Memorial Hospital for the purpose of developing and sustaining a primary care physician network in Eastern North Carolina. He was appointed to the latter position in July 1996, after having served as senior associate dean of the School of Medicine for the previous 5 years. He currently serves on a number of national advisory committees and boards, including the advisory committee for the Pew Foundation's Health Professions Schools in Service to America program. He lectures widely on the subject of the interface of health services education and service to rural and underserved populations, institutional change, physician leadership, and pediatric medicine.

Joyce C. Lashof, M.D., D.M.Sc. (Hon), is currently associate chair of the editorial board of the *UC Berkeley Wellness Letter* in the School of Public Health at the University of California, Berkeley. She is the former dean and professor emerita of the School of Public Health at the University of California, Berkeley. Previously, Dr. Lashof was assistant director of the congressional Office of Technology Assessment and earlier was director of the Illinois Department of Public Health. Dr. Lashof was president of the American Public Health Association, and she has been a member of several committees including the Medical Advisory Committee, the California Department of Health Services, the Health Care Financing Subcommittee of the Health Care and Public Policy Committee, and the American College of Physicians.

Patrick H. Mattingly, M.D., is a consultant in health care organization, strategy, and quality, with clients including the Agency on Health Care Research and Quality and the Picker Institute where he serves as a senior consultant. From 1993-1998, he was the senior vice president of planning and development at Harvard Pilgrim Health Care in Brookline, Massachusetts, and previously served as president and medical director of the Harvard Community Health Plan of New England in Providence, Rhode Island. Between 1981 and 1989, Dr. Mattingly served as president and chief executive officer of the Wyman Park Health System, an integrated health care system that merged into the Johns Hopkins Health System. From 1989 to 1990, Dr. Mattingly served as an Institute of Medicine scholar-in-residence with the Council on Health Care Technology and is a member of many professional organizations, including the Group Health Association of America and the American College of Physician Executives. Dr. Mattingly received his M.D. degree from Harvard Medical School.

Carolina Reyes, M.D., is associate director of the Division of Women's Health Policy and Research and a Maternal-Fetal Medicine attending physician in the Department of Obstetrics and Gynecology at Cedars-Sinai Medical Center. She is a visiting assistant professor in the Department of Obstetrics and Gynecology, University of California, Los Angeles School of Medicine. Dr. Reyes is a senior scholar with the Agency for Healthcare Research and Quality. Her research focuses on developing maternal quality indicators to better assess the quality of care provided to women. Dr. Reyes is the senior medical advisor for the National Alliance for Hispanic Health—the oldest and largest network of providers serving over 10 million Hispanics. She is an appointed member of the Secretary of Health's Advisory Committee on Infant Mortality. She received her Bachelor of Arts degree from Stanford University and her Medical Doctorate degree from Harvard Medical School.

Cheryl J. Roberts, J.D., is the director of managed care for the Virginia Department of Medical Assistance Services. In this capacity, Ms. Roberts is responsible for developing and implementing managed care, special needs, and quality assurance programs for the state's Medicaid managed care consumers. Ms. Roberts is a health insurance professional with 17 years of experience in developing health care initiatives in both the public and the private sectors. She served as assistant vice president of Group Health Inc., in New York, and chief operating officer of Virginia Chartered Health Plan, a Medicaid health maintenance organization. Ms. Roberts has developed physical and behavioral health programs as well as maternal child health programs. She currently serves on the Board of the Richmond Young Women's Christian Association. Ms. Roberts received her Juris Doctor from Rutgers University Law School in New Jersey.

Stephen A. Somers, Ph.D., is president and chief executive officer of the Center for Health Care Strategies, Inc. (CHCS), which he founded in 1995. CHCS is a nonprofit policy resource center dedicated to promoting the development and implementation of effective health policy for vulnerable Americans. It is affiliated with Princeton University's Woodrow Wilson School of Public and International Affairs, where Dr. Somers is a visiting lecturer and visiting senior research scholar. For the decade prior to establishing CHCS, Dr. Somers was an associate vice-president and a program officer at the Robert Wood Johnson Foundation. Dr. Somers is also director of the Foundation's Medicaid Managed Care Program and a senior consultant to the Building Health Systems for People with Chronic Illnesses Program. Dr. Somers has an extensive program management and health policy background. He holds a Ph.D. from Stanford University.

Ann Zuvekas, D.P.A., is a senior fellow at the Center for Health Services Research and Policy, School of Public Health and Health Services, The George Washington University Medical Center, as well as a private consultant. She has served as principal investigator and senior advisor on studies of patients' experiences in community and migrant health centers, the impact of managed care programs on safety net providers who serve vulnerable populations and on the populations themselves, hospital-primary care relationships, developing health status measures to evaluate primary health care for poor and minority Americans, evaluating options for the structure of the nation's poison control center system, and examining the causes of the low infant-mortality rate among persons of Mexican descent. Formerly, Dr. Zuvekas was a vice president at The Lewin Group. She received her D.P.A. in Health Services Administration and Public Administration from The George Washington University.

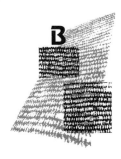

Workshop Agenda

INSTITUTE OF MEDICINE
Committee on the Changing Market, Managed Care, and the
Future Viability of Safety Net Providers
May 7–8, 1998

Atrium Ballroom, Washington Court Hotel
525 New Jersey Avenue, N.W., Washington, D.C.

THURSDAY, MAY 7, 1998

8:30 a.m. **Registration and Continental Breakfast**

9:00 a.m. **Welcome and Introductions**
Stuart Altman, Ph.D. (*Chair*)
Sol C. Chaikin Professor of National Health Policy
Heller Graduate School of Social Policy
Brandeis University

9:15–10:45 a.m. **Panel 1: The Status of Safety Net Providers: What Does the Research Tell Us?**
This session will explore the research and data collection activities currently being conducted by some of

the leading policy research organizations directed at assessing the changing environment and its impact on safety net providers.

Moderator: Raymond Baxter, Ph.D.
Senior Vice President
The Lewin Group

Peter Cunningham, Ph.D.
Senior Health Researcher
Center for Studying Health System Change

John Holahan, Ph.D.
Director, Health Policy Center
The Urban Institute

Robert Hurley, Ph.D.
Associate Professor
Department of Health Administration
Virginia Commonwealth University

Sara Rosenbaum, J.D.
Hirsh Professor of Health Care Law and Policy
Center for Health Policy Research
The George Washington University

10:45–12:15 p.m.   Panel 1 *continued*: Research Findings

Moderator: John Billings, J.D.
Associate Professor and Director of
Health Research Programs
Robert F. Wagner School of Public
Service
New York University

Joel Cantor, Sc.D.
Director of Research
United Hospital Fund

Suzanne Felt-Lisk, M.P.A.
Senior Researcher
Mathematica Policy Research, Inc.

Magda Peck, Sc.D.
Chief Executive Officer and Executive Director
CityMatCH
University of Nebraska Medical Center,
  Department of Pediatrics

Diane Rowland, Sc.D.
Senior Vice President
Commission on Medicaid and the Uninsured
Henry J. Kaiser Family Foundation

12:30–1:30 p.m.   **Lunch: Federal and State Perspectives on the Role of Safety Net Providers in the New Health Care Environment** (Atrium Ballroom)

Christine Ferguson, J.D.
Director
Rhode Island Department of Human Services
Cranston, Rhode Island

1:45–3:15 p.m.   **Panel 2: Provider Perspective**
This session will assess the impact that the changing health care market and the shift to Medicaid managed care is having on safety net providers. How are these changes affecting their funding streams, patient population, scope of services, and organizational structure? How are they affecting their ability to serve the uninsured and special needs populations? What are some of the lessons being learned regarding keys to survival and major obstacles?

Moderator: Thomas Irons, M.D.
Associate Vice Chancellor for Health
  Sciences
East Carolina University School of
  Medicine
President, Health East

Terry Conway, M.D.
Chief Medical Officer
Cooke County Bureau of Health Services

Marilyn Gaston, M.D.
Director, Bureau of Primary Care
Health Resources and Services Administration

Marla Gold, M.D.
Section Chief, HIV/AIDS Medicine
Allegheny University Hospitals-Hahnemann

Jane McCaleb, M.D.
Medical Director
Rural Health Group, Inc.

Cornell Scott, M.P.H.
Executive Director
Hill Health Corporation

3:15–3:30 p.m.   Break

**3:30–5:00 p.m.   Panel 3: Medicaid Managed Care and New Roles
and Responsibilities for Safety Net Providers:
Perspective of States, Local Agencies, Medicaid
Agencies, and MCOs**
This session will look at the impact of Medicaid managed care and other changes on safety net providers.

Moderator: Patrick Mattingly, M.D.
Senior Vice President
Planning and Development
Harvard Pilgrim Health Care

Mark Finucane
Director of Health Services
Los Angeles County Department of Health

Catherine Halverson
Vice President of Medicaid Programs
United Healthcare

Michael G. Lucas
Assistant Health Commissioner
Philadelphia Department of Public Health

Vernon K. Smith, Ph.D.
Principal
Health Management Associates

5:00 p.m.   **Adjourn for the day**

FRIDAY, MAY 8, 1998

8:00 a.m.   **Continental Breakfast and Registration**

8:30–10:00 a.m.   **Panel 4: Constituent/Advocate Perspective**
This will be an opportunity to hear from patients, providers, special populations, and advocate groups who have directly seen how the shift to managed care has affected vulnerable populations traditionally served by safety net providers.

Moderator: Stuart Altman, Ph.D.
Sol C. Chaikin Professor of National
    Health Policy
Heller Graduate School of Social Policy
Brandeis University

Jeff Crowley, M.P.H.
Associate Executive Director
National Association of People Living
    with HIV/AIDS

Adolph P. Falcón, M.P.P.
Vice President of Policy and Research
National Coalition of Hispanic Health
    and Human Services

Dara Howe
Tennessee Coordinator
Family Voices

10:00–10:15 a.m.   **Break**

10:15 a.m.–
12:30 p.m.

Public Hearing

This will also be an opportunity for pre-registered participants to present a public testimony for the record. Their comments will be limited to 5 to 10 minutes and will be followed by questions from the committee members.

Moderator: Stuart Altman, Ph.D.
Sol C. Chaikin Professor of National Health Policy
Heller Graduate School of Social Policy
Brandeis University

Allan S. Noonan, M.D., M.P.H.
Director
D.C. Department of Health
Association of State and Territorial Health Officials

Charles De Brunner
Executive Director
National Association of Urban Critical Access Hospitals

Charlotte Collins
Of Counsel
National Association of Public Hospitals and Health Systems

Daniel R. Hawkins, Jr.
Vice President for Federal and State Affairs
National Association of Community Health Centers

Catherine A. Hess, M.S.W.
Executive Director
Association of Maternal and Child Health Programs

Athol W. Morgan, M.D.
Cardiovascular Specialists of Maryland
Urban Medical Institute
Liberty Medical Center

Gregory Branch, M.D., CEO
Gerard Family Associates

Diane M. Becker, Sc.D., M.P.H.
Associate Professor of Medicine
Director, Center for Health Promotion
The Johns Hopkins University School of Medicine

12:30 p.m.   **Workshop Adjourns**

12:30–3:30 p.m.   **Committee Meets in Executive Session (closed to the public)**

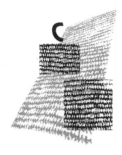

Workshop Participants

COMMITTEE MEMBERS

Stuart Altman, Ph.D.
Sol C. Chaikin Professor of
    National Health Policy
Heller Graduate School of Social
    Policy
Brandeis University
Waltham, MA

John Bartlett, M.D.
Chief, Division of Infectious
    Diseases
Johns Hopkins University School
    of Medicine
Baltimore, MD

Raymond Baxter, Ph.D.
Senior Vice President
The Lewin Group
Fairfax, VA

John Billings, Ph.D.
Associate Professor and Director
    of Health Research Programs
Robert F. Wagner School of Public
    Service
New York University
New York, NY

Donna Checkett*
Chief Executive Officer
Missouri Care Health Plan
Columbia, MO

Patricia A. Gabow, M.D.
CEO and Medical Director
Denver Health
Denver, CO

Mary L. Hennrich, R.N., M.S.
Chief Executive Officer
CareOregon
Portland, OR

---

*Resigned from committee August 5, 1998.

Sandral Hullett, M.D.
Executive Director
West Alabama Health Services,
    Inc.
Eutaw, AL

Tom Irons, M.D.
Associate Vice Chancellor for
    Health Services
President, Health East
Greenville, NC

Joyce C. Lashof, M.D.
Professor Emerita
School of Public Health
University of California at Berkeley
Berkeley, CA

Patrick Mattingly, M.D.
Senior Vice President
Planning and Development
Harvard Pilgrim Health Care
Brookline, MA

Carolina Reyes, M.D.
Assistant Professor
Obstetrics and Gynecology
The George Washington
    University Medical Center
Washington, DC

Cheryl J. Roberts, J.D.
Director of Managed Care
Virginia Department of Medical
    Assistance Services
Richmond, VA

Stephen Somers, Ph.D.
President
Center for Health Care Strategies,
    Inc.
Princeton, NJ

Ann Zuvekas, D.P.A.
Senior Research Staff Scientist
Center for Health Policy Research
The George Washington University
Washington, DC

PARTICIPANTS

Rhoda Abrams
Associate Bureau Director
Office of Program and Policy
    Development
Health Resources and Services
    Administration (HRSA)
Bethesda, MD

Tamara Allen
Program Analyst
HRSA/Center for Managed Care
Rockville, MD

Ann Calvaresi Barr
Senior Policy Analyst
U.S. General Accounting Office
Washington, DC

Diane M. Becker, Sc.D., M.P.H.
Associate Professor of Medicine
Director, Center for Health
    Promotion
The Johns Hopkins University
    School of Medicine
Baltimore, MD

Clyde J. Behney
Deputy Executive Officer
Institute of Medicine
Washington, DC

Amy Bernstein, Ph.D.
Senior Research Manager
The Alpha Center
Washington, DC

Cheryl Beversdorf, R.N., M.H.S.,
C.A.E.
Executive Vice President
Association of State and Territorial
Health Officials
Washington, DC

Gregory Branch, M.D.
Chief Executive Officer
Gerard Family Associates
Washington, DC

Fish Brown
Director of Public Policy
Catholic Health Association of the
U.S.
Washington, DC

Christine Burch
Executive Director
The National Association of Public
Hospitals and Health Systems
Washington, DC

Joel Cantor, Sc.D.
Director of Research
United Hospital Fund
New York, NY

K. Lynn Cates, M.D.
Robert Wood Johnson Health
Policy Fellow
Office of Senator James Jeffords
Senate Labor and Human
Resources Committee
Washington, DC

Carolyn Clancy, M.D.
Director, Center for Primary Care
Research
Agency for Health Care Policy
and Research
U.S. Dept. of Health and Human
Services (DHHS)
Rockville, MD

Melissa H. Clarke, M.P.A.
Health Care Policy and Program
Analyst
HRSA
Rockville, MD

Gary Claxton
Deputy Assistant Secretary for
Planning and Evaluation/
Health Policy
DHHS
Washington, DC

Charlotte Collins
Of Counsel
National Association of Public
Hospitals and Health Systems
Washington, DC

Barbara Cooper
Director
Office of Strategic Planning
Health Care Financing
Administration
Washington, DC

Peter Cunningham, Ph.D.
Senior Health Researcher
Center for Studying Health
System Change
Washington, DC

Charles DeBrunner
Executive Director
National Association of Urban
    Critical Access Hospitals
Washington, DC

Juliann DeStefano
Policy Analyst
Maternal and Child Health Bureau
HRSA
Rockville, MD

Anne Dievler, Ph.D.
Senior Policy Analyst
U.S. General Accounting Office
Washington, DC

Alden (Joe) Doolittle
Consultant
Center for Managed Care
HRSA
Rockville, MD

Jennifer Dunbar
Policy Analyst
Project Hope
Center for Health Affairs
Bethesda, MD

Catherine Dunham, Ed.D.
Program Director
Robert Wood Johnson Community
    Health Leadership Program
Boston, MA

Jeffrey D. Dunlap
Senior Analyst
HRSA/Office of Field
    Coordination
Rockville, MD

Brent Ewig
Associate Director for Access
    Policy
Association of State and Territorial
    Health Officials
Washington, DC

Adolph P. Falcón, M.P.P.
Vice President of Policy and
    Research
National Coalition of Hispanic
    Health and Human Services
Washington, DC

Suzanne Felt-Lisk, MPA
Senior Researcher
Mathematica Policy Research, Inc.
Washington, DC

Christine Ferguson
Director
Rhode Island Dept. of Human
    Services
Cranston, RI

Jennifer Fiedelholtz
Public Health Analyst
Office of Policy and Program
    Coordination
Substance Abuse and Mental
    Health Services
    Administration
Rockville, MD

Mark Finucane
Director of Health Services
Los Angeles County Department
    of Health
Los Angeles, CA

Darrell Gaskin, Ph.D.
Research Assistant Professor
Institute for Health Care Research
     and Policy
Georgetown University Medical
     Center
Washington, DC

Marilyn H. Gaston, M.D.
Director, Bureau of Primary
     Health Care
HRSA
Bethesda, MD

Marla J. Gold
Section Chief-HIV/AIDS Medicine
Allegheny University Hospitals-
     Hahnemann
Department of Medicine
Division of Infectious Diseases
Philadelphia, PA

Nanette Goodman
Policy Analyst
The National Association of Public
     Hospitals and Health Systems
Washington, DC

Katie-Louise Gottfried
Director, Primary Health and
     Managed Care Team
Office of Disease Prevention and
     Health Promotion
DHHS
Washington, DC

George Greenberg
Senior Advisor
Office of Health Policy
Assistant Secretary for Planning
     and Evaluation
DHHS
Washington, DC

Alison Hall
Program Officer
The Commonwealth Fund
New York, NY

Catherine Halverson
Vice President of Medicaid
     Programs
United Healthcare
Edina, MN

Dana Harchick
Fellowship Assistant
Association for Health Services
     Research
Washington, DC

Jeff Harris
Senior Policy Analyst
Health Policy Studies Division
National Governors' Association
Washington, DC

Dan Hawkins
Vice President for Federal and
     State Affairs
National Association of
     Community Health Centers
Washington, DC

Timothy Henderson, M.S.P.H.
Director, Primary Care Resource
     Center
National Conference of State
     Legislatures
Washington, DC

Tiffany Ho
Fellow
House Ways and Means
     Committee
Washington, DC

John Holahan, Ph.D.
Director, Health Policy Center
The Urban Institute
Washington, DC

Katie Horton
Professional Health Staff
Minority Senate Finance
    Committee
Washington, DC

Dara Howe
Tennessee State Coordinator
Family Voices
Tennessee Disability Coalition
Nashville, TN

Robert Hurley, Ph.D.
Associate Professor
Department of Health
    Administration
Medical College of Virginia/
    Virginia Commonwealth
    University
Richmond, VA

Ellen Hutchins, Sc.D.
Acting Chief, Perinatal and
    Women's Health Branch
Maternal and Child Health Bureau
Rockville, MD

David Introcaso
Vice President of Planning
DC General Hospital
Washington, DC

Sue Kaplan, J.D.
Associate Professor
New York University
New York, NY

Michele D. Kipke, Ph.D.
Director, Forum on Adolescence
Institute of Medicine
Washington, DC

Janet Kline
Specialist in Health Policy
Congressional Research Service
Washington, DC

Ellen Kugler
Associate Director
National Association of Urban
    Critical Access Hospitals
Washington, DC

Deborah Lamm, M.P.A.
Program Director
Community Health In Focus
Chevy Chase, MD

Bonnie Lefkowitz
Associate Bureau Director
Bureau of Primary Health Care
Bethesda, MD

Peter Levin, Ph.D.
Health Policy Counsel
Office of Senator Connie Mack
Washington, DC

Celia J. Maxwell, M.D., F.A.C.P.
Robert Wood Johnson Health
    Policy Fellow
Office of Senator Tom Harkin
Washington, DC

Jane McCaleb, M.D.
Medical Director
Rural Health Group, Inc.
Jackson, NC

James McClyde
Assistant Director, Health Services
     Quality and Public Health
U.S. General Accounting Office
Washington, DC

Bob McKay
Director, Housing and
     Homelessness
Child Welfare League of America
Washington, DC

Robert Mechanic
Senior Manager
The Lewin Group
Fairfax, VA

Mike L. Millman
Senior Staff Fellow
Office of Planning and
     Evaluation/HRSA
Rockville, MD

Judith D. Moore
Deputy Director, Center for
Medicaid and State Operations
Health Care Financing
     Administration
Baltimore, MD

Athol Morgan, M.D.
Cardiovascular Specialists of
     Maryland
Urban Medical Institute
Liberty Medical Center
Baltimore, MD

Jack Needleman, Ph.D.
Assistant Professor of Economics
     and Health Policy
School of Public Health
Harvard University
Cambridge, MA

Karen Nelson
Senior Health Specialist
Office of Congressman Henry A.
     Waxman
Washington, DC

Danielle Noll
Congressional Fellow
Congressman Pete Stark
Washington, DC

Allan S. Noonan, M.D., M.P.H.
Director
DC Department of Health
Washington, DC

Stephen Norton
Research Associate
The Urban Institute
Washington, DC

Tracey Orloff
Senior Policy Analyst
Health Policy Division
National Governors' Association
Washington, DC

Mary Jo O'Brien
Vice President
The Lewin Group
Fairfax, VA

Magda Peck, ScD
CEO and Executive Director
CityMatCH and Associate
     Chairperson for Community
     Health
University of Nebraska Medical
     Center
Department of Pediatrics
Omaha, NB

Gretchen Morley Rinne
Research Assistant
Health Research Program
New York, NY

Sara Rosenbaum, J.D.
Hirsh Professor of Health Care
    Law and Policy
Center for Health Policy Research
The George Washington
    University
Washington, DC

Alexander Ross, Sc.D.
Health Policy Analyst
Center for Managed Care/HRSA
Rockville, MD

Diane Rowland, Sc.D.
Senior Vice President
Commission on the Future of
    Medicaid
Henry J. Kaiser Family
    Foundation
Washington, DC

Cornell Scott, M.P.H.
Executive Director
Hill Health Center
New Haven, CT

Robert Seifert
Senior Policy Analyst
Robert Wood Johnson Community
    Health Leadership Program
Access Project
Boston, MA

Sandra Sherman
Assistant Director, Health Policy
American Medical Association
Washington, DC

Alexandra E. Shields, M.A.
Fellow
Institute for Health Policy
Florence Heller Graduate School
    for Advanced Studies in Social
    Welfare
Brandeis University
Waltham, MA

Janet L. Shikles, M.S.W.
Director of Public Policy and
    Government Relations
Powers, Pyles, Sutter, and Verville
International Square
Washington, DC

Harvey Sloane, M.D.
Senior Policy Advisor
U.S. Domestic Programs
Walsh Center for Rural Health
    Analysis
Bethesda, MD

Vernon K. Smith, Ph.D.
Principal
Health Management Associates
Lansing, MI

Helen L. Smits, M.D.
President and Medical Director
HealthRight, Inc.
Meriden, CT

Lynn Squire
Legislative Officer
Maternal and Child Health Bureau
Office of Program Development
Rockville, MD

Stephanie Talmadge
Public Health Analyst
HIV/AIDS Bureau/HRSA
Rockville, MD

Caroline Taplin
Senior Policy Analyst
Office of Health Policy
DHHS
Washington, DC

Kristin Testa
Legislative Health Staff
Senate Finance Committee,
    Minority Side
Washington, DC

Leigh Thurmond
Health Analyst
Bureau of Primary Health Care
Bethesda, MD

Jennifer Tolbert
Senior Financial/Policy Analyst
National Association of Public
    Hospitals and Health Systems
Washington, DC

Jessica Townsend
Senior Fellow Staff
HRSA
Rockville, MD

Margaret Trinity
Deputy Director
Public Programs
The American Association of
    Health Plans
Washington, DC

Jorge Velazquez
Special Assistant to the Assistant
    Secretary
DHHS
Administration for Children and
    Families
Washington, DC

Patricia Vinh-Thomas
Legislative Assistant
Senate Labor Committee, Minority
Washington, DC

Kathie Westpheling
Director of Organizational
    Relations
Association of Clinicians for the
    Underinsured
Vienna, VA

Tom Wildsmith
Policy Research Actuary
Health Insurance Association of
    America
Washington, DC

INSTITUTE OF MEDICINE STAFF

Marion Ein Lewin, M.A.
Senior Staff Officer and Director
Office of Health Policy Programs
    and Fellowships
Washington, DC

Justine Lang
Research Assistant
Office of Health Policy Programs
    and Fellowships
Washington, DC

Kari A. McFarlan
Administrative Assistant
Office of Health Policy Programs
    and Fellowships
Washington, DC

Cassandra T. Walker
Office of Health Policy Programs
    and Fellowships
Washington, DC

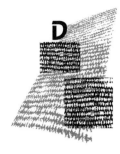

California Regional Meeting Agenda

MEDI-CAL POLICY INSTITUTE
and
INSTITUTE OF MEDICINE
Committee on the Changing Market, Managed Care, and the
Future Viability of Safety Net Providers
December 10, 1998

Oakland Marriott City Center
Oakland, CA

8:30 a.m.	Registration and Continental Breakfast
8:45 a.m.	Welcome and Introductions
9:00 a.m.	Overview of the Institute of Medicine Study
9:30 a.m.	Evidence and Perspectives from the California Market
12:00 p.m.	Lunch
1:30 p.m.	Lessons Learned: How Are Safety Net Providers Adapting to Survive Successfully in the New Environment?
3:30 p.m.	Closing Comments and Wrap-Up

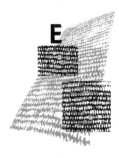

California Regional Meeting Participants

Rhoda Abrams
Associate Bureau for Policy
Office of Program and Policy
    Development
Bureau of Primary Health Care
Bethesda, MD

David F. Altman
Vice President
The Lewin Group
San Francisco, CA

Regina Aragon
Director for Public Policy
San Francisco AIDS Foundation
San Francisco, CA

Sharon Avery
Executive Director
Rural Healthcare Center
California Healthcare Association
Sacramento, CA

Raymond Baxter
Senior Vice President
The Lewin Group
Fairfax, VA

Mickie Beyer
Chief Executive Officer
Council of Community Clinics
San Diego, CA

John Billings
School of Public Service
New York University
New York, NY

Andrew B. Bindman, M.D.
Associate Professor of Medicine
UCSF Primary Care Research
    Center
San Francisco General Hospital
San Francisco, CA

Milton Camhi
Chief Executive Officer
Contra Costa Health Plan
Martinez, CA

Richard Chambers
Associate Regional Administrator
  for Medicaid
Health Care Financing
  Administration
San Francisco, CA

Carl E. Coan
President and Chief Executive
  Officer
Pediatric and Family Medical
  Center
Los Angeles, CA

Bob Derzon
Senior Vice President Emeritus
The Lewin Group
Mill Valley, CA

Mary K. Dewane
Chief Executive Officer
Executive Offices
CalOPTIMA
Orange, CA

Michael Dimmitt
California Healthcare Association
Sacramento, CA

Alicia Dixon
Program Director
Laurel Consulting Group
Los Angeles, CA

Jeanette Dong
Project Director
Asian Health Services
Community Voices
Oakland, CA

Ernestine Esparza
Executive Director
Vacaville Community Clinic
Vacaville, CA

Wendy Everette
Executive Director
Institute for the Future
Menlo Park, CA

Kathleen M. Eyre
Director, Government Affairs
The Permanente Medical Group
Oakland, CA

Leonard Finocchio
Associate Professor
UCSF Center for the Health
  Professions
San Francisco, CA

Lark Galloway-Gilliam
Executive Director
Administration
Community Health Councils, Inc.
Los Angeles, CA

Susanne Ginsburg
Vice President
The Lewin Group
San Francisco, CA

Ingrid Aguire Happoldt
Policy Analyst
Medi-Cal Policy Institute
Oakland, CA

Crystal Hayling
Director
Medi-Cal Policy Institute
Oakland, CA

James H. Hickman, Jr.
Director, Bay Area Region
Medi-Cal and Healthy Families
    Programs
Blue Cross of California
San Francisco, CA

Robert Isman, D.D.S., M.P.H.
Dental Program Consultant
Office of Medi-Cal Dental Services
California Department of Health
    Services
Sacramento, CA

Sylvia Drew Ivie
Executive Director
T.H.E. Clinic for Women, Inc.
Los Angeles, CA

Lucy Johns
Independent Consultant
Health Care Planning and Policy
San Francisco, CA

David B. Jomaoas
Director, Managed and
    Ambulatory Service
San Joaquin County Health Care
    Services
French Camp, CA

Adriene Josephs
Development Coordinator
San Francisco Community Clinic
    Corp.
San Francisco, CA

David J. Kears, M.S.W.
Director
Alameda County Health Care
    Services
San Leandro, CA

Jodi Korb
Senior Research Associate
Laguna Research Associates
San Francisco, CA

Joyce C. Lashof, M.D.
Professor Emerita
School of Public Health
University of California at
    Berkeley
Berkeley, CA

Marion Ein Lewin
Senior Staff Officer
IOM Safety Net Study
Institute of Medicine
Washington, DC

Valerie Lewis
Program Manager/Analyst
Medi-Cal Policy Institute
Oakland, CA

Susan Maerki, MHSA, MAE
SCM and Associates/RAND
    Consultant
San Francisco, CA

Burt Margolin
Director of Public Policy
Brady and Berliner Law Firm
Los Angeles, CA

Denise K. Martin, M.P.H.
President and Chief Executive
    Officer
California Association of Public
    Hospitals and Health
Berkeley, CA

Patrick Mattingly
Senior Vice President Planning
    and Development
Harvard Pilgrim Health Care
Brookline, CA

B. Kathlyn Mead
President and Chief Executive
    Officer
Sharp Health Plan
San Diego, CA

Randall Mecham
Special Projects Coordinator
Health and Human Services
    Agency
San Diego, CA

Ann Monroe
Quality Initiative
California Health Care Foundation
Oakland, CA

Kathleen Morkert
Director of Managed Care
Medical Management
Planned Parenthood Mar Monte
San Jose, CA

Leah Morris
Sr. Program Officer
Managed Care and Health Grants
Sierra Health Foundation
Sacramento, CA

Peter Nakahata
Director, Program Development
CalOPTIMA
Orange, CA

Claudia Page
Research Analyst
Medi-Cal Policy Institute
Oakland, CA

Timothy Reilly
Consultant
Pacific Health Consulting Group
San Anselmo, CA

Thomas Rundall
Professor
Health Policy and Management
University of California, Berkeley
Berkeley, CA

Alexandra Shields
Senior Research Associate
Institute for Health Care Research
Georgetown University
Washington, DC

Ralph Silber
Executive Director
Alameda Health Consortium
Oakland, CA

Robert Sillen
Executive Director,
    Administration
Santa Clara Valley Health and
    Hospital System
San Jose, CA

Cynthia Solomon
Chief Executive Officer
Medi-Cal Management Resources
Sonoma, CA

Herrmann Spetzler
Chief Executive Officer
Open Door Health Centers
Arcata, CA

Alan Stolmack
Chief, Plan Monitoring/Member
    Rights Branch
California Department of Health
    Services
Medi-Cal Managed Care Division
Sacramento, CA

Carrie Fletcher Stover
Asst. Director of Government
    Relations
The California Medical
    Association
Sacramento, CA

Lucy Street
Finance and Data Analyst
Medi-Cal Policy Institute
Oakland, CA

Robin Strimling
Health Insurance Specialist
Division of Medicaid
Health Care Financing
    Administration
San Francisco, CA

John Troidl
Consultant
Health Services Management
Davis, CA

Don Trujillo
Regional Advocate
California Primary Care
    Association
Sacramento, CA

Debra M. Ward
Vice President, External Affairs
External Affairs
Watts Health Systems, Inc./HP
    Healthcare
Inglewood, CA

Joanna K. Weinberg, JD, LLM
Associate Adjunct Professor
Institute for Health and Aging
Department of Social and
    Behavioral Sciences
University of California, San
    Francisco
San Francisco, CA

Lucien Wulsin, Jr.
Law Offices of Lucien Wulsin, Jr.
Santa Monica, CA

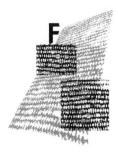 New York Regional Meeting Agenda

THE COMMONWEALTH FUND
and
INSTITUTE OF MEDICINE
The Changing Market, Managed Care, and the
Future Viability of Safety Net Providers
Wednesday, January 13, 1999

New York University's Lipton Hall, D'Agostino Hall
108 West Third Street, New York City

9:00 a.m.   **Registration and Continental Breakfast**

9:30 a.m.   **Welcome and Introduction**
Brian Biles
Senior Vice President
The Commonwealth Fund

Stuart Altman
Chair, IOM Study on the Changing Market, Managed
Care, and the Future Viability of Safety Net Providers
Sol C. Chaikin Professor of National Health Policy
Heller Graduate School of Social Policy
Brandeis University

9:35 a.m.   **Overview of New York Safety Net and Trends in**
Health Care Marketplace

Brief presentations
• Demand on the Safety Net
Kathryn Haslanger
Director of Policy Analysis
United Hospital Fund

• Structure of the Safety Net
Joel Cantor
Director of Research
United Hospital Fund

• Support for the Safety Net
Deborah Bachrach
Partner
Kalkines, Arky, Zall and Bernstein

Discussion

10:15 a.m.   **Medicaid Managed Care—The "Roll-Out" and Its**
Impact

Brief presentations
• A Brief History
Kathryn Haslanger
Director of Policy Analysis
United Hospital Fund

• Current Rate Structure
Patricia Kutel
Assistant Director, Office of Managed Care
Bureau of Managed Care Financing
New York State Department of Health

• Plan/Provider Perspective
Maura Bluestone
President and Chief Executive Officer
Bronx Health Plan

Discussion

11:15 a.m. **Graduate Medical Education and the Safety Net**

Brief presentations
• A Brief Overview
Pat Wang
Senior Vice President, Health Finance and
    Managed Care
Greater New York Hospital Association

• Community-Based Provider Perspective
Robert Massad
Chairman of Family Medicine
Montefiore Medical Center
Albert Einstein College of Medicine

Discussion

12:15 p.m. **Lunch**

1:15 p.m. **The Role of the Public Health Care Delivery System**

Brief presentations
Richard Langfelder
Senior Vice President, Finance
New York City Health and Hospitals Corporation

Charles Brecher
Professor
Robert F. Wagner Graduate School of Public Service
New York University

Discussion

2:00 p.m.   **Providing Direct Support for the Safety Net**

Brief presentations
Judy Arnold
Deputy Commissioner
Planning, Policy and Resource Development
New York State Department of Health

Ronda Kotelchuck
Executive Director
Primary Care Development Corporation

Discussion

3:00 p.m.   **Adjourn**

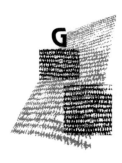

New York Regional Meeting Participants

COMMITTEE MEMBERS

Stuart Altman, Ph.D. (*Chair*)
Sol C. Chaikin Professor of
   National Health Policy
Heller Graduate School of Social
   Policy
Brandeis University
Waltham, MA

Raymond Baxter, Ph.D.
Senior Vice President
The Lewin Group
Fairfax, VA

John Billings, J.D.
Associate Professor and Director
   of Health Research Programs
Robert F. Wagner School of Public
   Service
New York University
New York, NY

Sandral Hullett, M.D.
Executive Director
West Alabama Health Services, Inc.
Eutaw, AL

Patrick Mattingly, M.D.
Senior Vice President
Planning and Development
Harvard Pilgrim Health Care
Brookline, MA

Stephen Somers, Ph.D.
President
Center for Health Care Strategies,
   Inc.
Princeton, NJ

253

PARTICIPANTS

Dennis P. Andrulis, Ph.D.
Head of the Office of Urban
   Populations
New York Academy of Medicine
New York, NY

Judith Arnold
Deputy Commissioner, Planning,
   Policy and Resource
   Development
New York State Department of
   Health
Albany, NY

Deborah Bachrach, Esq.
Partner
Kalkines, Arky, Zall and Bernstein
New York, NY

Julio Bellber
President and Chief Executive
   Officer
Center Care
New York, NY

Elisabeth Benjamin
Staff Attorney
Legal Aid
New York, NY

Alice Berger
Director, Health Care Planning
Planned Parenthood of New York
   City
New York, NY

Brian Biles, M.D., M.P.H.
Senior Vice President
The Commonwealth Fund
New York, NY

Leah F. Binder
Senior Project Advisor
Mayor's Office of Health Services
New York, NY

Maura Bluestone
President and CEO
Bronx Health Plan
Bronx, NY

Charles Brecher
Professor
Robert F. Wagner School of Public
   Service
New York University
New York, NY

Joel Cantor, Sc.D.
Director of Research
United Hospital Fund
New York, NY

James L. Capoziello
Deputy Commissioner
Division of Health Care Access
New York City Department of
   Health
New York, NY

Benjamin K. Chu, M.D., M.P.H.
Vice President of Clinical Affairs
   and Associate Dean
New York University Medical
   Center
New York, NY

Rima J. Cohen
Vice President, Insurance Options
Greater New York Hospital
   Association
New York, NY

Barry Ensminger
Executive Director
Planned Parenthood of New York
    City
New York, NY

Oliver Fein, M.D.
Associate Dean for Network
    Affairs
Weill Medical College of Cornell
    University
New York, NY

Herbert Fillmore, M.S.W.
Director of Research
Village Care of New York
New York, NY

Kristine Gebbie, M.N., Dr.P.H.
Elizabeth Standish Gill Associate
    Professor of Nursing and
Director, Center for Health Policy
    and Health Services Research
Columbia University; School of
    Nursing
New York, NY

H. Jack Geiger, M.D.
Arthur C. Logan Professor
    Emeritus
Department of Community Health
    and Social Medicine
City University of New York
    Medical School
New York, NY

Rosa M. Gil, DSW
Special Advisor to the Mayor for
    Health Policy
Mayor's Office of Health Services
New York, NY

Eli Ginzberg, Ph.D.
Director
Eisenhower Center for the
    Conservation of Human
    Resources
Columbia University
New York, NY

David Gould
Senior Vice President for
    Programs
United Hospital Fund
New York, NY

Bradford Gray
New York Academy of Medicine
New York, NY

Allyson Hall
Program Officer
The Commonwealth Fund
New York, New York

Kathryn Haslanger
Director of Policy Analysis
United Hospital Fund
New York, NY

Margaret C. Heagarty, M.D.
Director of Pediatrics
Columbia University Harlem
    Hospital Center and
Professor of Pediatrics
Columbia University College of
    Physicians and Surgeons
New York, NY

Karen Hein, M.D.
President
W.T. Grant Foundation
New York, NY

Allen I. Hyman, M.D., F.C.C.M.
Chief of Staff
New York Presbyterian Hospital
New York, NY

Ronda Kotelchuck
Executive Director
Primary Care Development
    Corporation
New York, NY

Patricia Kutel
Assistant Director
Office of Managed Care, Bureau of
    Managed Care Financing
New York State Department of
    Health
Albany, NY

Richard Langfelder
Senior Vice President, Finance
New York City Health and
    Hospitals Corporation
New York, NY

Joan M. Leiman
Executive Deputy Vice President
    for Health Sciences
Columbia University, College of
    Physicians and Surgeons
New York, NY

Sharon Lerner
Reporter
The Village Voice
New York, NY

Elizabeth Macfarlane
Director, Program Planning
Office of Managed Care
New York State Department of
    Health
Albany, NY

Robert Massad, M.D.
Chairman of Family Medicine
Montefiore Medical Center/Albert
    Einstein College of Medicine
Bronx, NY

Irwin R. Merkatz, M.D.
Professor and Chair
Department of Obstetrics and
    Gynecology and Women's
    Health
Vice President for Clinical
    Affiliations
Albert Einstein College of
    Medicine/Montefiore Medical
    Center
Bronx, NY

Julie Minter
Director, Office of Program
    Development and Evaluation
Department of Health, Division of
    Health Care Access
New York, NY

Maria K. Mitchell
President
AMDEC
New York, NY

Roger D. Platt, M.D.
Vice President
Mount Sinai Health System
The Mount Sinai Medical Center
New York, NY

Ellen Rautenberg
President and Chief Executive
    Officer
Medical and Health Research
    Association of NYC, Inc.
New York, NY

Alexander F. Ross, Sc.D.
Health Policy Analyst
Center for Managed Care
Health Resources and Services
    Administration
Rockville, MD

David Sandman
Program Officer
The Commonwealth Fund
New York, NY

Denise Soffel, Ph.D.
Senior Policy Analyst, Health
Department of Public Policy
Community Service Society of
    New York
New York, NY

Joseph Sullivan
Chairman
Catholic Medical Center of
    Brooklyn and Queens
Brooklyn, NY

Raymond Sweeney
Executive Vice President
Health Care Association of New
    York State
Albany, NY

James R. Tallon, Jr.
President
United Hospital Fund
New York, NY

Lorraine Tregde
Consultant
Cathedral High School
Medical Gateway Department
New York, NY

Bruce C. Vladeck, Ph.D.
Professor of Health Policy
Mt. Sinai School of Medicine
New York, NY

Patricia Wang, Esq.
Senior Vice President, Health
    Finance and Managed Care
Greater New York Hospital
    Association
New York, NY

Judy Wessler
Policy Coordinator
Commission on the Public's
    Health System
New York, NY

STAFF

Marion Ein Lewin
Senior Staff Officer and Director
Office of Health Policy Programs
    and Fellowships
Institute of Medicine
Washington, DC

Judy Krauss
IOM/AAN Distinguished Senior
    Nurse Scholar-in-Residence
Office of Health Policy Programs
    and Fellowships
Institute of Medicine
Washington, DC

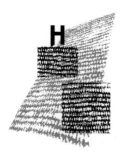

Rural Conference Call Participants

INSTITUTE OF MEDICINE
Committee on the Changing Market, Managed Care, and the
Future Viability of Safety Net Providers
October 7, 1998

Rural Safety Net Provider Issues

Rhoda Abrams, Associate Bureau Director, Office of Program and
Policy Development, Health Resources and Services Administration

Dr. Forest Calico, President, Appalachian Regional Healthcare

Tom Harward, Physician Assistant, Belington, West Virginia

Dr. Tom Irons, Associate Vice Chancellor for Health Sciences, East
Carolina University School of Medicine and President, Health East
(Institute of Medicine Committee Member)

Dr. Richard Kozoll, Physician, Cuba, New Mexico

Justine Lang, Research Assistant, Institute of Medicine

Marion Ein Lewin, Senior Staff Officer and Study Director, Institute of Medicine

Tom Morris, Policy Analyst, Office of Rural Health Policy, Health Resources and Services Administration

Tom Ricketts, Deputy Director, Cecil G. Sheps Center for Health Services Research (co-author of commissioned paper)

Alex Ross, Health Policy Analyst, Center for Managed Care, Health Resources and Services Administration

Becky Slifkin, Senior Research Associate and Director of Program on Health Care Economics and Finance, Cecil G. Sheps Center for Health Services Research (co-author of commissioned paper)

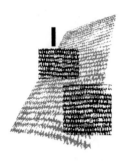

Acronyms

ACG	Ambulatory Care Group
ADA	Americans with Disabilities Act
AFDC	Aid to Families with Dependent Children
AHA	American Hospital Association
AHC	academic health center
AIDS	acquired immune deficiency syndrome
AMA	American Medical Association
AMC	academic medical center
BBA	Balanced Budget Act
CAHP	Consumer Assessment of Health Plans
CBO	Congressional Budget Office
CHC	community health center
CHPW	Community Health Plan of Washington
CPS	Current Population Survey
CSHSC	Center for Studying Health System Change
DHHS	U.S. Department of Health and Human Services
DSH	disproportionate share hospital
EPSDT	Early and Periodic Screening, Diagnosis, and Treatment
FQHC	federally qualified health center

GME	graduate medical education
HCFA	Health Care Financing Administration
HIPAA	Health Insurance Portability and Accountability Act
HIV	human immunodeficiency virus
HMO	health maintenance organization
HRSA	Health Resources and Services Administration
ICHD	Ingham County Health Department
IHS	Indian Health Service
IOM	Institute of Medicine
LACDHS	Los Angeles County Department of Health Services
LHD	local health department
MCHB	Maternal and Child Health Bureau
MCO	managed care organization
MedPAC	Medicare Payment Advisory Commission
MSA	medical savings account
MUA	medically underserved area
NAPH	National Association of Public Hospitals and Health Systems
NHC	Neighborhood Health Center
NHP	Neighborhood Health Plan
OBRA	Omnibus Budget Reconciliation Act
OCHD	Onondaga County Health Department
OHP	Oregon Health Plan
PCCM	primary care case management
PCDC	Primary Care Development Corporation
POS	point-of-service plan
PRWORA	Personal Responsibility and Work Opportunity Reconciliation Act
PSO	provider sponsored organization
RHC	rural health clinic
RHCG	Rural Health Care Group
SCHIP	State Children's Health Insurance Program
SLIPA	supplementary low-income patient adjustment
SMI	serious mental illness

SNOPAC	Safety Net Organizations and Patient Advisory Commission
SSDI	Social Security Disability Insurance
SSI	Supplemental Security Income
STD	sexually transmitted disease
TANF	Temporary Assistance to Needy Families
UDS	Uniform Data System
VA	Veterans Affairs
VHA	Veterans Health Administration
WIC	Special Supplemental Nutrition Program for Women, Infants, and Children

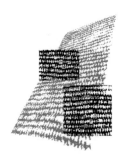

Index

A

Academic health centers, 48, 66, 83, 111, 148-149, 195, 209
Academic medical centers, 4, 23, 24, 56, 65-66, 72, 84, 114, 116-117, 135, 145, 146, 148-149, 161
Accessibility, health care, 1, 3, 4, 8, 10, 21, 27, 74, 175
  beneficiary choice, 7, 25, 30, 83-84, 166-170, 206-207; *see also* *"mainstreaming" infra*
  commercial *vs* Medicaid managed care, 161
  community funding, 13, 14
  community health centers, 59-60
  cost sharing/out-of-plan decisions, 32-33
  emergency care, 36
  local health departments, 63
  mainstreaming, 26, 30, 38-39, 135, 170-173, 176, 195
  Medicaid managed care, 161, 162-164, 170-173
  nonfinancial barriers, 166
    cultural factors, 21, 24, 41, 60, 159
    language barriers, 21, 24, 41, 48, 52, 53, 59, 73
  telephone access, 14, 161, 217
  transportation to care, 7, 21, 48, 56, 59, 137, 161, 163, 166, 185, 197
  outreach, 7, 13, 34, 48, 51, 57, 61, 74, 95, 97, 109, 166, 168, 208
    special-needs patients, 181, 195, 197, 198, 199, 218
  primary care, 7, 164
  primary care case management, 31-32, 139, 148, 149, 150, 162-163
  private practitioners, 162
  special-needs patients, 13, 51, 195, 197, 198, 199, 218
    outreach, 181, 195, 197, 198, 199, 218
  see also Advocacy; Core safety net providers; Insurance; Uninsured/underinsured persons
Accountability, 11, 136, 214
  community services funding, 13
  Medicaid, 29, 107, 133
  special-needs patients, 199, 201
Administrative requirements
  community health centers, 63, 102(n.25)
  cost-based reimbursement, 102(n.25)